ADHD

A Comprehensive Guide to Understanding, Diagnosis, and Treatment

Ethan D. Anderson

Xspurts.com

A New Zealand Designed Product

Other Versions Available

Why limit yourself to just one format?

This book is now available in physical, digital, and audiobook options.

Choose the way you love to read and dive into the story today. You won't regret it!

Digital ISBN: 9781776969258
Physical ISBN: 9781776969241
Audio ISBN:

To obtain a different format of this book at a discounted price, please get in touch with us at:

http://isbn.xspurts.com/

Contents

Have Questions / Comments?

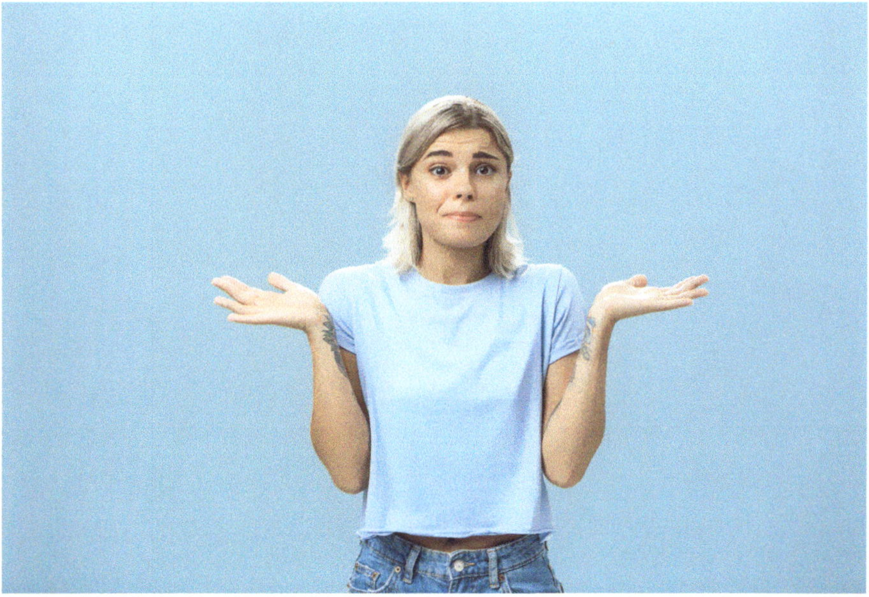

This book was designed to cover as much information as possible, but I know I have probably missed something, or some new amazing discovery has just come out.

If you notice something missing or have a question that I failed to answer, please get in touch and let me know. If I can, I will email you an answer and also update the book so others can also benefit from it.

Thanks For Being Awesome :)

Submit Your Questions / Comments At:

https://questions.xspurts.com

Get Free Stuff

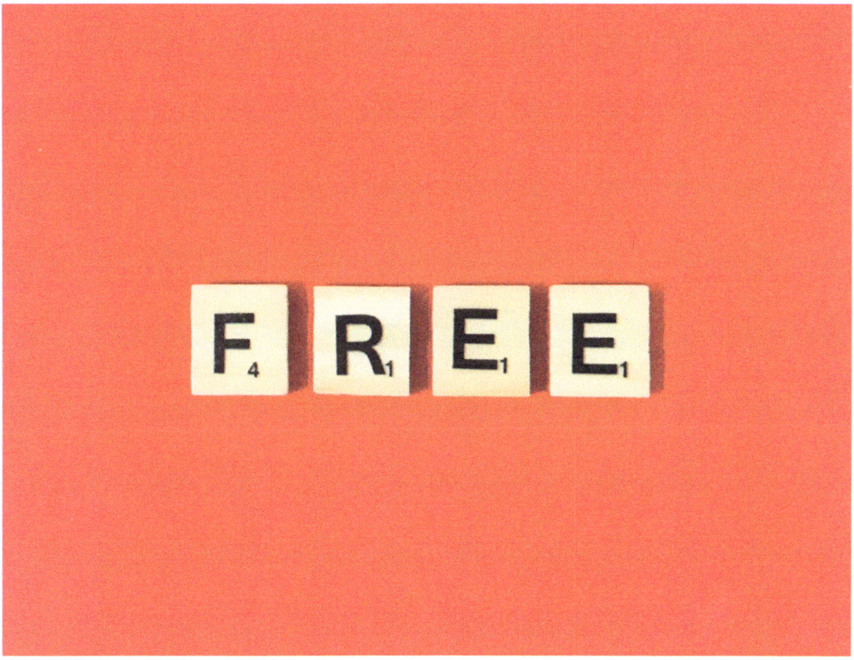

We love writing and have produced a huge number of books.

For being one of our amazing readers, we would love to offer you more books we have created, 100% free.

To claim this limited time special offer, simply go to the site below and enter your name and email address.

You will then receive loads (as we love our readers so much :) of our great books, content and audio direct to your email account, 100% free!

Get Loads of FREE Stuff at:

https://free.xspurts.com

Chapter One

Understanding ADHD

Attention Deficit Hyperactivity Disorder (ADHD) is a neurodevelopmental disorder that affects both children and adults. It is characterized by inattention, hyperactivity, and impulsivity, which can lead to academic, social, and occupational difficulties. ADHD is estimated to affect between 5-10% of children and approximately 2-5% of adults worldwide. Below we will we will explore the causes, symptoms, diagnosis, and treatment of ADHD.

Causes of ADHD

The exact cause of ADHD is unknown, but research suggests that it is a combination of genetic and environmental factors. Studies have shown that genetics play a significant role in the development of ADHD. It is estimated that up to 80% of ADHD cases have a genetic component. Several genes have been identified that are associated with the development of ADHD. Environmental factors such as exposure to toxins, premature birth, and maternal smoking during pregnancy have also been linked to ADHD.

Symptoms of ADHD

1. The symptoms of ADHD can be divided into three categories: inattention, hyperactivity, and impulsivity. Inattention symptoms include difficulty paying attention, forgetfulness, and being easily distracted. Hyperactivity symptoms include fidgeting, excessive talking, and difficulty sitting

still. Impulsivity symptoms include acting without thinking, interrupting others, and difficulty waiting their turn.

Diagnosis of ADHD

Diagnosing ADHD can be challenging as there is no specific test to diagnose it. A diagnosis of ADHD is usually made by a healthcare professional after a thorough assessment of the individual's symptoms and medical history. The assessment may include interviews with the individual, their family, and teachers, as well as standardized rating scales. The Diagnostic and Statistical Manual of Mental Disorders (DSM-5) is the most commonly used tool for diagnosing ADHD.

Treatment of ADHD

The treatment of ADHD typically involves a combination of medication and behavioral therapy. Stimulant medications such as methylphenidate and amphetamines are commonly used to treat ADHD. These medications work by increasing the levels of neurotransmitters in the brain that are responsible for regulating attention and behavior. Behavioral therapy can help individuals with ADHD learn coping strategies, improve their social skills, and manage their symptoms. Parent training and education can also be beneficial for children with ADHD.

Alternative treatments such as dietary changes, supplements, and exercise have also been studied for their effectiveness in treating ADHD. Some studies have suggested that a diet low in processed foods and high in omega-3 fatty acids can be beneficial for individuals with ADHD. Supplements such as zinc, iron, and magnesium have also been studied for their potential benefits. Exercise has been shown to improve cognitive function and behavior in individuals with ADHD.

Impact of ADHD

ADHD can have a significant impact on an individual's academic, social, and occupational functioning. Children with ADHD may struggle in school due to their difficulty with attention and organization. They may also have difficulty making and maintaining friendships due to their impulsivity and hyperactivity. Adults with ADHD may struggle with organization, time management, and completing tasks at work. They may also have difficulty maintaining relationships due to their impulsivity and forgetfulness.

In conclusion, ADHD is a neurodevelopmental disorder that affects both children and adults. It is characterized by inattention, hyperactivity, and impulsivity, which can lead to academic, social, and occupational difficulties. The exact cause of ADHD is unknown, but research suggests that it is a combination of genetic and environmental factors. Diagnosing ADHD can be challenging, and a diagnosis is usually made by a healthcare professional after a thorough assessment of the individual's symptoms and medical history. The treatment of ADHD typically involves a combination of medication and behavioral therapy. ADHD can have a significant impact on an individual's academic, social, and occupational functioning.

Definition, symptoms, and types of ADHD

ADHD, or Attention Deficit Hyperactivity Disorder, is a neurodevelopmental condition that can impact both children and adults. It is marked by symptoms such as inattention, hyperactivity, and impulsivity, which can lead to academic, social, and occupational difficulties. Below we will we will explore the definition, symptoms, and types of ADHD.

Definition of ADHD

ADHD is a disorder that affects the way the brain processes information. It is a developmental disorder that typically appears in childhood, although it can also be diagnosed in adulthood. Individuals with ADHD may have difficulty with attention, impulse control, and hyperactivity, which can impact their ability to function effectively in everyday life.

Symptoms of ADHD

1. The symptoms of ADHD can be divided into three categories: inattention, hyperactivity, and impulsivity.

Inattention symptoms include:

Difficulty paying attention to details or may make careless mistakes

Difficulty sustaining attention on tasks or activities

Difficulty listening when spoken to directly

Difficulty following through on instructions or completing tasks

Difficulty organizing tasks and activities

Avoidance or dislike of tasks that require sustained mental effort

Losing things necessary for tasks or activities

Forgetfulness in daily activities

Hyperactivity symptoms include:

Fidgeting with hands or feet or squirming in seat

Leaving seat in situations when remaining seated is expected

Running or climbing excessively in inappropriate situations

Difficulty playing or engaging in leisure activities quietly

Being "on the go" or acting as if "driven by a motor"

Talking excessively

Impulsivity symptoms include:

Acting without thinking

Blurting out answers before questions have been completed

Difficulty waiting their turn

Interrupting or intruding on others' conversations or activities

Types of ADHD

2. ADHD can be classified into three types based on the predominant symptoms: predominantly inattentive type, predominantly hyperactive-impulsive type, and combined type.

Predominantly Inattentive Type:

Individuals with this type of ADHD have symptoms of inattention but do not have significant hyperactivity or impulsivity. They may appear to be "daydreamers" or have trouble completing tasks due to their difficulty sustaining attention.

Predominantly Hyperactive-Impulsive Type:

Individuals with this type of ADHD have symptoms of hyperactivity and impulsivity but do not have significant problems with attention. They may appear to be restless or have difficulty sitting still.

Combined Type:

Individuals with this type of ADHD have symptoms of both inattention and hyperactivity-impulsivity. This is the most common type of ADHD.

Diagnosis of ADHD

Diagnosing ADHD can be challenging as there is no specific test to diagnose it. A diagnosis of ADHD is usually made by a healthcare professional after a thorough assessment of the individual's symptoms and medical history. The assessment may include interviews with the individual, their family, and teachers, as well as standardized rating scales. The Diagnostic and Statistical Manual of Mental Disorders (DSM-5) is the most commonly used tool for diagnosing ADHD.

Treatment of ADHD

The treatment of ADHD typically involves a combination of medication and behavioral therapy. Stimulant medications such as methylphenidate and amphetamines are commonly used to treat ADHD. These medications work by increasing the levels of neurotransmitters in the brain that are responsible for regulating attention and behavior. Behavioral therapy can help individuals with ADHD learn coping strategies, improve their social skills, and manage their symptoms. Parent training and education can also be beneficial for children with ADHD.

Alternative treatments such as dietary changes, supplements, and exercise have also been studied for their effectiveness in treating ADHD. Some studies have suggested that a diet low in processed foods and high in omega-3 fatty acids can be beneficial for individuals with ADHD. Supplements such as zinc, iron, and magnesium have also

The history and evolution of ADHD diagnosis

Attention Deficit Hyperactivity Disorder (ADHD) is a neurodevelopmental disorder that affects both children and adults. It is characterized by inattention, hyperactivity, and impulsivity, which can lead to academic, social, and occupational difficulties. Below we will we will explore the history and evolution of ADHD diagnosis.

History of ADHD Diagnosis

The symptoms of ADHD have been described in medical literature for over a century. In 1902, British pediatrician Sir George Frederic Still described a group of children who exhibited symptoms of restlessness, inattention, and impulsivity. He referred to this condition as "defective moral control."

In the 1930s and 1940s, several researchers described a condition known as "minimal brain dysfunction." This condition was characterized by symptoms of hyperactivity, impulsivity, and inattention. However, it was not until the 1960s that the term "hyperkinetic impulse disorder" was first used to describe the symptoms of ADHD.

The term "attention deficit disorder" (ADD) was first used in 1980 when the American Psychiatric Association (APA) included it in the third edition of the Diagnostic and Statistical Manual of Mental Disorders (DSM-III). This condition was characterized by symptoms of inattention but did not include hyperactivity or impulsivity.

In 1987, the APA revised the diagnostic criteria for ADD to include the symptoms of hyperactivity and impulsivity. The term "ADHD" was first used in the fourth edition of the DSM (DSM-IV) published in 1994.

Evolution of ADHD Diagnosis

1. The diagnostic criteria for ADHD have evolved over time. The DSM-IV identified three subtypes of ADHD: predominantly inattentive type, predominantly hyperactive-impulsive type, and combined type.

In 2013, the fifth edition of the DSM (DSM-5) was published. The diagnostic criteria for ADHD were revised to include several changes. The subtypes of ADHD were eliminated, and a single diagnosis of ADHD was established. The DSM-5 also lowered the age of onset for ADHD from 7 to 12 years old, reflecting the fact that symptoms can appear in younger children.

The DSM-5 also added new criteria for the diagnosis of ADHD. For example, individuals must now exhibit symptoms of inattention and/or hyperactivity-impulsivity before the age of 12. Additionally, the symptoms must be present in two or more settings (e.g., home, school, work) and must negatively impact academic, social, or occupational functioning.

Controversies in ADHD Diagnosis

The diagnosis of ADHD is not without controversy. Some critics argue that the diagnosis of ADHD is overused and that the symptoms are not specific to ADHD but can be found in other conditions such as anxiety or depression.

Others argue that the diagnostic criteria for ADHD are too broad and that many children who do not have ADHD are being diagnosed and treated unnecessarily with stimulant medications. There is also concern that stimulant medications such as methylphenidate and amphetamines can be abused and have potential long-term side effects.

However, proponents of ADHD diagnosis argue that it is a legitimate condition that can cause significant impairment in academic, social, and occupational functioning. They argue that appropriate diagnosis and treatment can improve outcomes for individuals with ADHD.

In conclusion, the history and evolution of ADHD diagnosis have been characterized by changing diagnostic criteria and controversy. The symptoms of ADHD have been described in medical literature for over a century, and the diagnostic criteria have evolved over time. The DSM-5 provides the current diagnostic criteria for ADHD, which includes a single diagnosis and the requirement of symptoms in two or more settings that impact academic, social, or occupational functioning. While the diagnosis of ADHD is not without controversy, proponents argue that appropriate

The role of genetics and environmental factors

Attention Deficit Hyperactivity Disorder (ADHD) is a neurodevelopmental disorder that affects both children and adults. It is characterized by inattention, hyperactivity, and impulsivity, which can lead to academic, social, and occupational difficulties. Below we will we will explore the role of genetics and environmental factors in the development of ADHD.

Genetics and ADHD

The exact cause of ADHD is unknown, but research suggests that genetics play a significant role in its development. It is estimated that up to 80% of ADHD cases have a genetic component.

Several genes have been identified that are associated with the development of ADHD. These genes are involved in the regulation of neurotransmitters in the brain, particularly dopamine and norepinephrine. These neurotransmitters are responsible for regulating attention, behavior, and motivation.

Research has also shown that ADHD is more common in families with a history of the disorder. Studies have found that the risk of developing ADHD is approximately four to five times higher if a first-degree relative such as a parent or sibling has the disorder.

Environmental Factors and ADHD

In addition to genetics, environmental factors such as prenatal exposure to toxins, premature birth, and maternal smoking during pregnancy have also been linked to ADHD.

Prenatal Exposure to Toxins:

Exposure to toxins such as lead, mercury, and polychlorinated biphenyls (PCBs) during pregnancy has been linked to an increased risk of ADHD. These toxins can cross the placenta and affect the developing fetal brain, leading to changes in brain structure and function that can contribute to ADHD.

Premature Birth:

Premature birth, or birth before 37 weeks of gestation, has been associated with an increased risk of ADHD. This may be due to the fact that premature infants are more vulnerable to brain injury and developmental problems.

Maternal Smoking during Pregnancy:

Maternal smoking during pregnancy has also been linked to an increased risk of ADHD. Nicotine and other chemicals in tobacco smoke can cross the placenta and affect the developing fetal brain, leading to changes in brain structure and function that can contribute to ADHD.

Other environmental factors that have been studied for their potential link to ADHD include low birth weight, maternal stress during pregnancy, and exposure to pesticides and other environmental toxins.

Interaction between Genetics and Environmental Factors

It is likely that the development of ADHD is the result of an interaction between genetics and environmental factors. For example, a child with a genetic predisposition to ADHD may be more vulnerable to the effects of prenatal exposure to toxins or maternal smoking during pregnancy.

Studies have also shown that environmental factors can modify the expression of genes associated with ADHD. For example, exposure to stress during pregnancy has been shown to increase the expression of genes associated with ADHD.

In conclusion, the role of genetics and environmental factors in the development of ADHD is complex. While genetics play a significant role in the development of ADHD, environmental factors such as prenatal exposure to toxins, premature birth, and maternal smoking during pregnancy have also been linked to an increased risk of the disorder. It is likely that the development of ADHD is the result of an interaction between genetics and environmental factors. Further research is needed to better understand the complex interplay between genetics and environmental factors in the development of ADHD.

Chapter Two

Diagnosis and Assessment

Attention Deficit Hyperactivity Disorder (ADHD) is a neurodevelopmental disorder that affects both children and adults. It is characterized by inattention, hyperactivity, and impulsivity, which can lead to academic, social, and occupational difficulties. Below we will we will explore the diagnosis and assessment of ADHD.

Diagnosis of ADHD

Diagnosing ADHD can be challenging as there is no specific test to diagnose it. A diagnosis of ADHD is usually made by a healthcare professional after a thorough assessment of the individual's symptoms and medical history. The assessment may include interviews with the individual, their family, and teachers, as well as standardized rating scales. The Diagnostic and Statistical Manual of Mental Disorders (DSM-5) is the most commonly used tool for diagnosing ADHD.

The DSM-5 provides the following diagnostic criteria for ADHD:

Inattention:

Difficulty paying attention to details or making careless mistakes

Difficulty sustaining attention on tasks or activities

Difficulty listening when spoken to directly

Difficulty following through on instructions or completing tasks

Difficulty organizing tasks and activities

Avoidance or dislike of tasks that require sustained mental effort

Losing things necessary for tasks or activities

Forgetfulness in daily activities

Hyperactivity:

Fidgeting with hands or feet or squirming in seat

Leaving seat in situations when remaining seated is expected

Running or climbing excessively in inappropriate situations

Difficulty playing or engaging in leisure activities quietly

Being "on the go" or acting as if "driven by a motor"

Talking excessively

Impulsivity:

Acting without thinking

Blurting out answers before questions have been completed

Difficulty waiting their turn

Interrupting or intruding on others' conversations or activities

To meet the diagnostic criteria for ADHD, an individual must exhibit six or more symptoms of inattention and/or hyperactivity-impulsivity for at least six months. Additionally, the symptoms must be present before the age of 12 and must negatively impact academic, social, or occupational functioning.

Assessment of ADHD

Assessment of ADHD typically involves a comprehensive evaluation of the individual's symptoms and medical history. The assessment may include interviews with the individual, their family, and teachers, as well as standardized rating scales.

Standardized rating scales are often used to assess the severity of ADHD symptoms. These scales ask the individual, family members, and teachers to rate the individual's behavior on a scale from "never" to "very often." The results are then used to assess the severity of the individual's symptoms and to monitor treatment progress.

In addition to rating scales, neuropsychological testing may be used to assess cognitive function and identify any areas of weakness that may contribute to ADHD symptoms. This testing may include measures of attention, memory, and executive function.

Assessment of ADHD may also include a physical exam and laboratory testing to rule out any underlying medical conditions that may be contributing to the individual's symptoms. For example, thyroid disorders or sleep disorders can cause symptoms that mimic ADHD.

In conclusion, the diagnosis and assessment of ADHD involve a comprehensive evaluation of the individual's symptoms and medical history. A diagnosis of ADHD is typically made by a healthcare professional after a thorough assessment of the individual's symptoms and medical history, and the use of standardized rating scales. Assessment of ADHD may also include neuropsychological testing, a physical exam, and laboratory testing to rule out any underlying medical conditions that may be contributing to the individual's symptoms.

The process of diagnosing ADHD in children and adults

Attention Deficit Hyperactivity Disorder (ADHD) is a neurodevelopmental disorder that affects both children and adults. It is characterized by inattention, hyperactivity, and impulsivity, which can lead to academic, social, and occupational difficulties. Below we will we will explore the process of diagnosing ADHD in children and adults.

Diagnosing ADHD in Children

Diagnosing ADHD in children can be challenging as the symptoms of ADHD can overlap with typical childhood behavior. A diagnosis of ADHD is usually made by a healthcare professional after a thorough assessment of the child's symptoms and medical history. The assessment may include interviews with the child, their parents, and teachers, as well as standardized rating scales. The Diagnostic and Statistical Manual of Mental Disorders (DSM-5) is the most commonly used tool for diagnosing ADHD.

The DSM-5 provides the following diagnostic criteria for ADHD:

Inattention:

Difficulty paying attention to details or making careless mistakes

Difficulty sustaining attention on tasks or activities

Difficulty listening when spoken to directly

Difficulty following through on instructions or completing tasks

Difficulty organizing tasks and activities

Avoidance or dislike of tasks that require sustained mental effort

Losing things necessary for tasks or activities

Forgetfulness in daily activities

Hyperactivity:

Fidgeting with hands or feet or squirming in seat

Leaving seat in situations when remaining seated is expected

Running or climbing excessively in inappropriate situations

Difficulty playing or engaging in leisure activities quietly

Being "on the go" or acting as if "driven by a motor"

Talking excessively

Impulsivity:

Acting without thinking

Blurting out answers before questions have been completed

Difficulty waiting their turn

Interrupting or intruding on others' conversations or activities

To meet the diagnostic criteria for ADHD, a child must exhibit six or more symptoms of inattention and/or hyperactivity-impulsivity for at least six months. Additionally, the symptoms must be present before the age of 12 and must negatively impact academic, social, or occupational functioning.

Assessing ADHD in Children

Assessing ADHD in children typically involves a comprehensive evaluation of the child's symptoms and medical history. The assessment may include interviews with the child, their parents, and teachers, as well as standardized rating scales.

Standardized rating scales are often used to assess the severity of ADHD symptoms. These scales ask the child, parents, and teachers to rate the child's behavior on a scale from "never" to "very often." The results are then used to assess the severity of the child's symptoms and to monitor treatment progress.

In addition to rating scales, neuropsychological testing may be used to assess cognitive function and identify any areas of weakness that may contribute to ADHD symptoms. This testing may include measures of attention, memory, and executive function.

Assessing ADHD in children may also include a physical exam and laboratory testing to rule out any underlying medical conditions that may be contributing to the child's symptoms. For example, thyroid disorders or sleep disorders can cause symptoms that mimic ADHD.

Diagnosing ADHD in Adults

Diagnosing ADHD in adults can also be challenging as the symptoms of ADHD can overlap with other conditions such as anxiety and depression. A diagnosis of ADHD is usually made by a healthcare professional after a thorough assessment of the adult's symptoms and medical history. The assessment may include interviews with the adult, their family, and colleagues, as well as standardized rating scales. The DSM-5 is also used to diagnose ADHD in adults.

Assessment tools and criteria for diagnosis

Attention Deficit Hyperactivity Disorder (ADHD) is a neurodevelopmental disorder that affects both children and adults. It is characterized by inattention, hyperactivity, and impulsivity, which can lead to academic, social, and occupational difficulties. Below we will we will explore the assessment tools and criteria for the diagnosis of ADHD.

Assessment Tools for ADHD

There are several assessment tools that can be used to help diagnose ADHD. These tools are designed to gather information about an individual's symptoms and behaviors, and can be completed by the individual, their parents, and/or their teachers. The following are some of the most commonly used assessment tools for ADHD:

1. Conners' Rating Scales: The Conners' Rating Scales are a series of rating scales that are used to assess the severity of ADHD symptoms. The scales include questions about the individual's behavior and are completed by the individual, their parents, and teachers.

2. Vanderbilt Assessment Scales: The Vanderbilt Assessment Scales are a series of rating scales that are used to assess the severity of ADHD symptoms. The scales include questions about the individual's behavior and are completed by the individual, their parents, and teachers.

3. Barkley Adult ADHD Rating Scale: The Barkley Adult ADHD Rating Scale is a self-report questionnaire that is designed to assess the severity of ADHD symptoms in adults.

4. Behavior Assessment System for Children: The Behavior Assessment System for Children is a comprehensive assessment tool that is used to assess a wide range of behavioral and emotional problems in children. The tool includes questions about the individual's behavior and is completed by the individual, their parents, and teachers.

5. Neuropsychological Testing: Neuropsychological testing can be used to assess cognitive function and identify any areas of weakness that may

contribute to ADHD symptoms. This testing may include measures of attention, memory, and executive function.

Diagnostic Criteria for ADHD

The Diagnostic and Statistical Manual of Mental Disorders (DSM-5) is the most commonly used tool for diagnosing ADHD. The DSM-5 provides the following diagnostic criteria for ADHD:

Inattention:

Difficulty paying attention to details or making careless mistakes

Difficulty sustaining attention on tasks or activities

Difficulty listening when spoken to directly

Difficulty following through on instructions or completing tasks

Difficulty organizing tasks and activities

Avoidance or dislike of tasks that require sustained mental effort

Losing things necessary for tasks or activities

Forgetfulness in daily activities

Hyperactivity:

Fidgeting with hands or feet or squirming in seat

Leaving seat in situations when remaining seated is expected

Running or climbing excessively in inappropriate situations

Difficulty playing or engaging in leisure activities quietly

Being "on the go" or acting as if "driven by a motor"

Talking excessively

Impulsivity:

Acting without thinking

Blurting out answers before questions have been completed

Difficulty waiting their turn

Interrupting or intruding on others' conversations or activities

To meet the diagnostic criteria for ADHD, an individual must exhibit six or more symptoms of inattention and/or hyperactivity-impulsivity for at least six months. Additionally, the symptoms must be present before the age of 12 and must negatively impact academic, social, or occupational functioning.

In conclusion, assessment tools and criteria are essential for the diagnosis of ADHD. There are several assessment tools available that can help gather information about an individual's symptoms and behaviors. The DSM-5 provides diagnostic criteria for ADHD that can be used to determine whether an individual meets the criteria for a diagnosis of ADHD. It is important for healthcare professionals to use a comprehensive assessment approach when diagnosing ADHD, which may include interviews with the individual, their parents, and teachers, as well as standardized rating scales and

Differentiating ADHD from other conditions

Attention Deficit Hyperactivity Disorder (ADHD) is a neurodevelopmental disorder that can be challenging to diagnose, as its symptoms can overlap with other conditions. It is essential for healthcare professionals to differentiate ADHD from other conditions to ensure that individuals receive the appropriate treatment. Below we will we will explore how ADHD can be differentiated from other conditions.

Differentiating ADHD from Anxiety Disorders

Anxiety disorders, such as generalized anxiety disorder and social anxiety disorder, can present with symptoms that are similar to those of ADHD. Both conditions can lead to difficulty concentrating, restlessness, and irritability. However, individuals with anxiety disorders may also experience excessive worry, fear, and panic attacks. Additionally, anxiety disorders can cause physical symptoms such as sweating, trembling, and heart palpitations.

To differentiate ADHD from anxiety disorders, healthcare professionals may use rating scales that specifically assess symptoms of anxiety. They may also ask the individual about the onset and duration of symptoms, as anxiety symptoms typically occur in response to specific situations, whereas ADHD symptoms are present in multiple settings.

Differentiating ADHD from Depression

Depression can also present with symptoms that are similar to those of ADHD, such as difficulty concentrating, irritability, and fatigue. However, individuals with depression may also experience feelings of sadness, hopelessness, and worthlessness. Additionally, depression can cause physical symptoms such as changes in appetite and sleep patterns.

To differentiate ADHD from depression, healthcare professionals may use rating scales that specifically assess symptoms of depression. They may also ask the individual about the onset and duration of symptoms, as depression symptoms typically occur for extended periods, whereas ADHD symptoms are present for at least six months.

Differentiating ADHD from Autism Spectrum Disorder

Autism Spectrum Disorder (ASD) can present with symptoms that are similar to those of ADHD, such as difficulty with social interactions and communication. However, individuals with ASD may also exhibit restricted, repetitive behaviors and interests. Additionally, individuals with ASD may not understand social cues, such as facial expressions and body language.

To differentiate ADHD from ASD, healthcare professionals may use rating scales that specifically assess symptoms of ASD. They may also ask the individual about their social interactions and communication abilities.

Differentiating ADHD from Learning Disabilities

Learning disabilities, such as dyslexia and dyscalculia, can present with symptoms that are similar to those of ADHD, such as difficulty with attention and organization. However, individuals with learning disabilities may also experience difficulty with reading, writing, and math skills.

To differentiate ADHD from learning disabilities, healthcare professionals may use neuropsychological testing to assess cognitive function and identify any areas of weakness that may contribute to symptoms. They may also ask the individual about their academic performance and any difficulties they may have had in school.

In conclusion, differentiating ADHD from other conditions can be challenging as its symptoms can overlap with other conditions. It is important for healthcare professionals to use a comprehensive assessment approach when evaluating individuals for ADHD, which may include interviews with the individual, their parents, and teachers, as well as standardized rating scales and neuropsychological testing. By differentiating ADHD from other conditions, healthcare professionals can ensure that individuals receive the appropriate treatment and support.

Chapter Three

ADHD and Coexisting Conditions

Attention Deficit Hyperactivity Disorder (ADHD) is a neurodevelopmental disorder that can coexist with other conditions. It is important to identify and address coexisting conditions in individuals with ADHD, as they can impact treatment and outcomes. Below we will we will explore some of the most common coexisting conditions that occur with ADHD.

Oppositional Defiant Disorder (ODD)

Oppositional Defiant Disorder (ODD) is a behavioral disorder that is characterized by defiant and disobedient behavior, often directed toward authority figures. ODD is estimated to occur in up to 50% of individuals with ADHD.

Symptoms of ODD include:

Frequent temper tantrums

Arguing with authority figures

Refusing to comply with rules and requests

Deliberately annoying others

Blaming others for mistakes

Being easily annoyed or angered

Being spiteful or vindictive

To address ODD in individuals with ADHD, a behavioral intervention program may be implemented, which may include parent training, behavior modification, and cognitive-behavioral therapy.

Anxiety Disorders

Anxiety disorders, such as generalized anxiety disorder and social anxiety disorder, are estimated to occur in up to 30% of individuals with ADHD. Anxiety disorders can impact academic and social functioning and can exacerbate ADHD symptoms.

Symptoms of anxiety disorders include:

Excessive worry

Fear and panic attacks

Avoidance of social situations

Physical symptoms such as sweating, trembling, and heart palpitations

To address anxiety disorders in individuals with ADHD, a combination of medication and therapy may be used. Cognitive-behavioral therapy and exposure therapy are effective treatments for anxiety disorders.

Depression

Depression is estimated to occur in up to 30% of individuals with ADHD. Depression can cause feelings of sadness, hopelessness, and worthlessness, and can exacerbate ADHD symptoms.

Symptoms of depression include:

Feelings of sadness and hopelessness

Loss of interest in activities

Changes in appetite and sleep patterns

Fatigue and low energy

Difficulty concentrating

To address depression in individuals with ADHD, a combination of medication and therapy may be used. Cognitive-behavioral therapy and interpersonal therapy are effective treatments for depression.

Learning Disabilities

Learning disabilities, such as dyslexia and dyscalculia, are estimated to occur in up to 40% of individuals with ADHD. Learning disabilities can impact academic functioning and can exacerbate ADHD symptoms.

Symptoms of learning disabilities include:

Difficulty with reading, writing, and math skills

Difficulty with attention and organization

Difficulty with executive function skills

To address learning disabilities in individuals with ADHD, educational interventions may be used, such as individualized education plans (IEPs) and 504 plans.

In conclusion, coexisting conditions are common in individuals with ADHD and can impact treatment and outcomes. It is important to identify and address coexisting conditions in individuals with ADHD to ensure that they receive the appropriate treatment and support. Behavioral interventions, medication, and therapy are effective treatments for coexisting conditions, and a comprehensive approach to treatment can improve outcomes for individuals with ADHD.

Common comorbid disorders with ADHD

Attention Deficit Hyperactivity Disorder (ADHD) is a neurodevelopmental disorder that can often coexist with other disorders. These comorbid conditions can impact the presentation, diagnosis, and treatment of ADHD. Below we will we will explore some of the most common comorbid disorders with ADHD.

Anxiety Disorders

Anxiety disorders, such as Generalized Anxiety Disorder (GAD) and Social Anxiety Disorder (SAD), are common comorbid disorders with ADHD. The prevalence of anxiety disorders in individuals with ADHD is estimated to be between 20-30%.

Symptoms of anxiety disorders include excessive worry, fear, and panic attacks. Individuals with anxiety disorders may also experience physical symptoms such as sweating, trembling, and heart palpitations. These symptoms can exacerbate ADHD symptoms such as restlessness, irritability, and difficulty concentrating.

Treatment for comorbid anxiety disorders and ADHD often includes a combination of medication and therapy. Cognitive-behavioral therapy (CBT) and exposure therapy are effective treatments for anxiety disorders.

Mood Disorders

Mood disorders, such as depression and bipolar disorder, are also common comorbid disorders with ADHD. The prevalence of mood disorders in individuals with ADHD is estimated to be between 20-30%.

Symptoms of mood disorders include feelings of sadness, hopelessness, and worthlessness. Individuals with mood disorders may also experience changes in appetite and sleep patterns, fatigue, and difficulty concentrating. These symptoms can exacerbate ADHD symptoms such as impulsivity and distractibility.

Treatment for comorbid mood disorders and ADHD often includes a combination of medication and therapy. CBT and interpersonal therapy are effective treatments for depression, while medication and psychotherapy are effective treatments for bipolar disorder.

Oppositional Defiant Disorder (ODD)

Oppositional Defiant Disorder (ODD) is a behavioral disorder that is characterized by defiant and disobedient behavior, often directed toward authority figures. The prevalence of ODD in individuals with ADHD is estimated to be between 30-50%.

Symptoms of ODD include frequent temper tantrums, arguing with authority figures, refusing to comply with rules and requests, and being easily annoyed or angered. These symptoms can exacerbate ADHD symptoms such as impulsivity and hyperactivity.

Treatment for comorbid ODD and ADHD often includes a behavioral intervention program that may include parent training, behavior modification, and CBT.

Substance Use Disorders

Substance use disorders, such as alcohol and drug addiction, are also common comorbid disorders with ADHD. The prevalence of substance use disorders in individuals with ADHD is estimated to be between 20-30%.

Symptoms of substance use disorders include the use of substances despite negative consequences, withdrawal symptoms, and an inability to stop using. These symptoms can exacerbate ADHD symptoms such as impulsivity and poor judgment.

Treatment for comorbid substance use disorders and ADHD often includes a combination of medication and therapy. Cognitive-behavioral therapy and motivational interviewing are effective treatments for substance use disorders.

In conclusion, comorbid disorders are common in individuals with ADHD and can impact the presentation, diagnosis, and treatment of ADHD. Anxiety disorders, mood disorders, oppositional defiant disorder, and substance use disorders are some of the most common comorbid disorders with ADHD. A comprehensive approach to treatment that addresses comorbid disorders can improve outcomes for individuals with ADHD.

The impact of coexisting conditions on ADHD management

Attention Deficit Hyperactivity Disorder (ADHD) is a neurodevelopmental disorder that can often coexist with other conditions. These coexisting conditions can impact the management of ADHD, including diagnosis, treatment, and outcomes. Below we will we will explore the impact of coexisting conditions on ADHD management.

Diagnosis

The presence of coexisting conditions can complicate the diagnosis of ADHD. For example, symptoms of anxiety and depression can overlap with symptoms of ADHD, making it difficult to distinguish between the two disorders. Additionally, symptoms of oppositional defiant disorder and conduct disorder can exacerbate ADHD symptoms, making it difficult to determine whether the behavior is due to ADHD or the coexisting disorder.

To ensure an accurate diagnosis, healthcare professionals must conduct a comprehensive evaluation that considers the presence of coexisting conditions. This evaluation may include interviews with the individual, their parents, and teachers, as well as standardized rating scales and neuropsychological testing.

Treatment

The presence of coexisting conditions can impact the management of ADHD. For example, individuals with ADHD and anxiety may require medication and therapy to address both conditions. If anxiety is left untreated, it can exacerbate ADHD symptoms such as restlessness, irritability, and difficulty concentrating.

Additionally, the presence of coexisting conditions can impact medication management. For example, individuals with ADHD and bipolar disorder may require different medications than individuals with ADHD alone. Healthcare professionals must consider the potential interactions between medications and the potential side effects when prescribing medications for individuals with coexisting conditions.

Outcomes

The presence of coexisting conditions can impact outcomes for individuals with ADHD. For example, individuals with ADHD and anxiety may experience greater academic and social impairment than individuals with ADHD alone. Similarly, individuals with ADHD and depression may have poorer treatment outcomes than individuals with ADHD alone.

Additionally, the presence of coexisting conditions can impact the long-term outcomes for individuals with ADHD. For example, individuals with ADHD and substance use disorders may be at higher risk for legal and financial problems, as well as poor academic and vocational outcomes.

To improve outcomes for individuals with ADHD and coexisting conditions, healthcare professionals must use a comprehensive treatment approach that addresses both disorders. This approach may include medication, therapy, and behavioral interventions, as well as support for academic and vocational success.

In conclusion, the presence of coexisting conditions can impact the management of ADHD, including diagnosis, treatment, and outcomes. Healthcare professionals must consider the potential impact of coexisting conditions when evaluating and treating individuals with ADHD. By using a comprehensive treatment approach that addresses both ADHD and coexisting conditions, healthcare professionals can improve outcomes for individuals with ADHD.

Strategies for managing multiple diagnoses

Managing multiple diagnoses can be challenging for both healthcare professionals and individuals with ADHD. Coexisting conditions such as anxiety disorders, mood disorders, oppositional defiant disorder, and substance use disorders can impact the management of ADHD. Below we will we will explore strategies for managing multiple diagnoses in individuals with ADHD.

Comprehensive Evaluation

The first step in managing multiple diagnoses in individuals with ADHD is to conduct a comprehensive evaluation that considers the presence of coexisting conditions. This evaluation should include interviews with the individual, their parents, and teachers, as well as standardized rating scales and neuropsychological testing.

By conducting a comprehensive evaluation, healthcare professionals can identify the presence of coexisting conditions and develop an individualized treatment plan that addresses both ADHD and the coexisting condition.

Collaborative Care

Collaborative care is an approach to healthcare that involves a team of healthcare professionals working together to provide coordinated care. This approach is particularly effective for individuals with multiple diagnoses, as it allows healthcare professionals to address the unique needs of each individual.

For example, a team of healthcare professionals may include a psychiatrist, a therapist, a pediatrician, and a special education teacher. By working together, these professionals can provide medication management, therapy, academic support, and behavioral interventions.

Medication Management

Medication management is an important aspect of managing multiple diagnoses in individuals with ADHD. Healthcare professionals must consider the potential interactions between medications and the potential side effects when prescribing medications for individuals with coexisting conditions.

Additionally, healthcare professionals must consider the potential for medication misuse and abuse, particularly in individuals with ADHD and substance use disorders. Regular monitoring and drug testing may be necessary to ensure safe medication use.

Cognitive-Behavioral Therapy (CBT)

Cognitive-behavioral therapy (CBT) is an effective treatment for both ADHD and many coexisting conditions, including anxiety disorders and mood disorders. CBT is a form of talk therapy that focuses on identifying and changing negative thought patterns and behaviors.

CBT can be adapted to address the unique needs of individuals with multiple diagnoses. For example, CBT may include exposure therapy for individuals with anxiety disorders or interpersonal therapy for individuals with mood disorders.

Behavioral Interventions

Behavioral interventions, such as parent training and behavior modification, are effective treatments for oppositional defiant disorder and conduct disorder. These interventions focus on teaching parents and caregivers strategies for managing challenging behavior, such as setting clear expectations and consequences.

Behavioral interventions may also include social skills training, which can improve the social functioning of individuals with ADHD and coexisting conditions.

Conclusion

In conclusion, managing multiple diagnoses in individuals with ADHD requires a comprehensive approach that addresses both ADHD and the coexisting condition. Strategies for managing multiple diagnoses include conducting a comprehensive evaluation, collaborative care, medication management, CBT, and behavioral interventions. By using a comprehensive approach to treatment, healthcare professionals can improve outcomes for individuals with ADHD and coexisting conditions.

Chapter Four

ADHD Medications

Attention Deficit Hyperactivity Disorder (ADHD) is a neurodevelopmental disorder that can be treated with medication. Medication can improve the symptoms of ADHD, including inattention, hyperactivity, and impulsivity. Below we will we will explore the medications used to treat ADHD.

Stimulants

Stimulant medications are the most commonly prescribed medications for ADHD. These medications work by increasing the levels of dopamine and norepinephrine in the brain, which can improve attention, concentration, and impulse control.

Stimulant medications include methylphenidate (Ritalin, Concerta, Daytrana) and amphetamine (Adderall, Vyvanse). These medications are available in immediate-release and extended-release formulations.

Stimulant medications can have side effects, including appetite suppression, weight loss, and sleep disturbances. These side effects are generally mild and can be managed by adjusting the dosage or switching to a different medication.

Non-Stimulants

Non-stimulant medications are an alternative to stimulant medications for individuals who do not respond well to or cannot tolerate stimulant medications. Non-stimulant medications work by increasing the levels of norepinephrine in the brain.

Non-stimulant medications include atomoxetine (Strattera), guanfacine (Intuniv), and clonidine (Kapvay). These medications are available in extended-release formulations.

Non-stimulant medications can have side effects, including nausea, vomiting, and dizziness. These side effects are generally mild and can be managed by adjusting the dosage or switching to a different medication.

Combination Therapy

Combination therapy involves the use of both stimulant and non-stimulant medications. Combination therapy may be effective for individuals who do not respond well to or cannot tolerate monotherapy.

Combination therapy can have side effects, including an increased risk of side effects associated with each medication. Healthcare professionals must carefully monitor individuals on combination therapy to ensure safe and effective treatment.

Lifestyle Changes

In addition to medication, lifestyle changes can also improve the symptoms of ADHD. These changes include:

1. Exercise: Regular exercise can improve attention, mood, and overall health.

2. Sleep: Adequate sleep is important for individuals with ADHD. Healthcare professionals may recommend sleep hygiene strategies or medications to improve sleep.

3. Diet: A healthy diet that includes a variety of nutrient-dense foods can improve overall health and cognitive function.

4. Behavioral Interventions: Behavioral interventions, such as parent training and behavior modification, can improve the social and behavioral functioning of individuals with ADHD.

Conclusion

In conclusion, medication can be an effective treatment for ADHD. Stimulant medications and non-stimulant medications are the most commonly prescribed medications for ADHD. Combination therapy and lifestyle changes can also improve the symptoms of ADHD. Healthcare professionals must carefully monitor individuals on medication to ensure safe and effective treatment. Additionally, lifestyle changes and behavioral interventions can be used in conjunction with medication to improve outcomes for individuals with ADHD.

Stimulant and non-stimulant medications for ADHD

1. Attention Deficit Hyperactivity Disorder (ADHD) is a neurodevelopmental disorder that can be treated with medications. There are two types of medications used to treat ADHD: stimulant and non-stimulant medications. Below we will we will explore the differences between these two types of medications and how they are used to treat ADHD.

Stimulant Medications

Stimulant medications are the most commonly prescribed medications for ADHD. These medications work by increasing the levels of dopamine and norepinephrine in the brain, which can improve attention, concentration, and impulse control.

Stimulant medications are available in immediate-release and extended-release formulations. Immediate-release formulations are taken two to three times a day and provide symptom relief for four to six hours. Extended-release formulations are taken once a day and provide symptom relief for up to 12 hours.

Stimulant medications include methylphenidate (Ritalin, Concerta, Daytrana) and amphetamine (Adderall, Vyvanse). These medications are available in different forms, including tablets, capsules, and patches.

Side effects of stimulant medications can include appetite suppression, weight loss, and sleep disturbances. These side effects are generally mild and can be managed by adjusting the dosage or switching to a different medication.

Non-Stimulant Medications

Non-stimulant medications are an alternative to stimulant medications for individuals who do not respond well to or cannot tolerate stimulant medications. Non-stimulant medications work by increasing the levels of norepinephrine in the brain.

Non-stimulant medications include atomoxetine (Strattera), guanfacine (Intuniv), and clonidine (Kapvay). These medications are available in extended-release formulations.

Side effects of non-stimulant medications can include nausea, vomiting, and dizziness. These side effects are generally mild and can be managed by adjusting the dosage or switching to a different medication.

Combination Therapy

Combination therapy involves the use of both stimulant and non-stimulant medications. Combination therapy may be effective for individuals who do not respond well to or cannot tolerate monotherapy.

Combination therapy can have side effects, including an increased risk of side effects associated with each medication. Healthcare professionals must carefully monitor individuals on combination therapy to ensure safe and effective treatment.

Which Medication is Right for You?

The decision to use stimulant or non-stimulant medication for ADHD depends on a number of factors, including the individual's age, medical history, and response to medication. Healthcare professionals must carefully evaluate each individual and develop an individualized treatment plan.

In general, stimulant medications are the first-line treatment for ADHD due to their effectiveness and rapid onset of action. Non-stimulant medications may be used in individuals who do not respond well to or cannot tolerate stimulant medications.

Conclusion

In conclusion, stimulant and non-stimulant medications are both effective treatments for ADHD. Stimulant medications increase the levels of dopamine and norepinephrine in the brain, while non-stimulant medications increase the levels of norepinephrine in the brain. Combination therapy may be effective for individuals who do not respond well to or cannot tolerate monotherapy. The decision to use stimulant or non-stimulant medication for ADHD depends on a number of factors and must be carefully evaluated by healthcare professionals.

How medications work and potential side effects

1. Medications are an important treatment option for individuals with Attention Deficit Hyperactivity Disorder (ADHD). There are two types of medications used to treat ADHD: stimulant and non-stimulant medications. Below we will we will explore how these medications work and their potential side effects.

How Medications Work

Stimulant Medications

Stimulant medications work by increasing the levels of dopamine and norepinephrine in the brain. These neurotransmitters are involved in the regulation of attention, concentration, and impulse control. By increasing the levels of dopamine and norepinephrine in the brain, stimulant medications can improve the symptoms of ADHD.

Stimulant medications are available in immediate-release and extended-release formulations. Immediate-release formulations are taken two to three times a day and provide symptom relief for four to six hours. Extended-release formulations are taken once a day and provide symptom relief for up to 12 hours.

Stimulant medications include methylphenidate (Ritalin, Concerta, Daytrana) and amphetamine (Adderall, Vyvanse). These medications are available in different forms, including tablets, capsules, and patches.

Non-Stimulant Medications

Non-stimulant medications work by increasing the levels of norepinephrine in the brain. Norepinephrine is involved in the regulation of attention and impulse control. By increasing the levels of norepinephrine in the brain, non-stimulant medications can improve the symptoms of ADHD.

Non-stimulant medications include atomoxetine (Strattera), guanfacine (Intuniv), and clonidine (Kapvay). These medications are available in extended-release formulations.

Potential Side Effects

Stimulant Medications

Stimulant medications can have side effects, including:

2. Appetite suppression: Stimulant medications can decrease appetite, leading to weight loss.

3. Sleep disturbances: Stimulant medications can interfere with sleep, leading to insomnia or disrupted sleep patterns.

4. Emotional lability: Stimulant medications can cause emotional changes, including irritability, mood swings, and anxiety.

5. Tics: Stimulant medications can exacerbate or cause tics.

6. Cardiovascular effects: Stimulant medications can cause an increase in heart rate and blood pressure.

7. Substance abuse: Stimulant medications can be misused or abused, leading to addiction or other substance use disorders.

Non-Stimulant Medications

Non-stimulant medications can have side effects, including:

8. Nausea and vomiting: Non-stimulant medications can cause gastrointestinal upset.

9. Dizziness: Non-stimulant medications can cause dizziness or lightheadedness.

10. Sedation: Non-stimulant medications can cause drowsiness or sedation.

11. Cardiovascular effects: Non-stimulant medications can cause an increase in heart rate and blood pressure.

12. Liver function: Non-stimulant medications can impact liver function and require monitoring.

Conclusion

In conclusion, medications are an important treatment option for individuals with ADHD. Stimulant medications work by increasing the levels of dopamine and norepinephrine in the brain, while non-stimulant medications work by increasing the levels of norepinephrine in the brain. Stimulant and non-stimulant medications can have potential side effects, including appetite suppression, sleep disturbances, emotional lability, tics, cardiovascular effects, and substance abuse for stimulant medications and nausea and vomiting, dizziness, sedation, cardiovascular effects, and liver function for non-stimulant medications. Healthcare professionals must carefully monitor individuals on medication to ensure safe and effective treatment.

The process of finding the right medication and dosage

Attention Deficit Hyperactivity Disorder (ADHD) is a neurodevelopmental disorder that can be treated with medication. The process of finding the right medication and dosage for individuals with ADHD can be complex and requires careful evaluation by healthcare professionals. Below we will we will explore the process of finding the right medication and dosage for ADHD.

1. Step 1: Evaluation

The first step in finding the right medication and dosage for ADHD is evaluation. Healthcare professionals must carefully evaluate each individual and develop an individualized treatment plan.

Evaluation includes a comprehensive medical history, physical examination, and assessment of ADHD symptoms. Healthcare professionals may also use standardized rating scales to assess the severity of ADHD symptoms.

In addition to evaluating ADHD symptoms, healthcare professionals must also evaluate coexisting conditions, including anxiety, depression, and substance use disorders. These coexisting conditions can impact treatment options and outcomes.

2. Step 2: Medication Selection

Once an individual has been evaluated, healthcare professionals can select a medication based on the individual's medical history, physical examination, and assessment of ADHD symptoms.

Stimulant medications are the first-line treatment for ADHD due to their effectiveness and rapid onset of action. Non-stimulant medications may be used in individuals who do not respond well to or cannot tolerate stimulant medications.

The selection of medication also depends on the individual's age, medical history, and potential side effects. Healthcare professionals must carefully weigh the potential benefits and risks of each medication.

3. Step 3: Initial Dosage

Once a medication has been selected, healthcare professionals will start with an initial dosage. The initial dosage is generally low and gradually increased over time to achieve the desired therapeutic effect.

Stimulant medications are available in immediate-release and extended-release formulations. Immediate-release formulations are taken two to three times a day and provide symptom relief for four to six hours. Extended-release formulations are taken once a day and provide symptom relief for up to 12 hours.

Non-stimulant medications are available in extended-release formulations and are generally taken once a day.

4. Step 4: Monitoring

After starting medication, healthcare professionals must carefully monitor the individual's response to medication and adjust the dosage as needed. The goal is to achieve the maximum therapeutic effect with the minimum effective dosage.

Monitoring includes regular follow-up appointments, standardized rating scales to assess symptom severity, and evaluation of potential side effects. Healthcare professionals must carefully weigh the potential benefits and risks of each medication and dosage.

5. Step 5: Adjustment

If the initial medication and dosage are not effective or cause side effects, healthcare professionals may adjust the medication or dosage. Adjustment may involve switching to a different medication or adjusting the dosage of the current medication.

Healthcare professionals must carefully evaluate each individual and develop an individualized treatment plan. The process of finding the right medication and dosage for ADHD can take time and requires careful monitoring and evaluation.

Conclusion

In conclusion, the process of finding the right medication and dosage for ADHD requires careful evaluation, medication selection, initial dosage, monitoring, and adjustment. Healthcare professionals must carefully evaluate each individual and develop an individualized treatment plan. Stimulant medications are the first-line treatment for ADHD, and non-stimulant medications may be used in individuals who do not respond well to or cannot tolerate stimulant medications. The goal is to achieve the maximum therapeutic effect with the minimum effective dosage while monitoring potential side effects. The process of finding the right medication and dosage for ADHD can take time and requires careful monitoring and evaluation by healthcare professionals.

Chapter Five

Behavioral Therapies and Interventions

Attention Deficit Hyperactivity Disorder (ADHD) is a neurodevelopmental disorder that can be treated with behavioral therapies and interventions. These treatments focus on improving social, emotional, and academic functioning and can be used alone or in combination with medication. Below we will we will explore the different types of behavioral therapies and interventions for ADHD.

Behavioral Therapy

Behavioral therapy is a form of psychotherapy that focuses on changing behavior. Behavioral therapy for ADHD aims to improve social, emotional, and academic functioning by teaching individuals with ADHD new skills and strategies.

Behavioral therapy for ADHD includes the following:

1. Parent Training: Parent training involves teaching parents how to manage their child's behavior and develop a positive relationship with their child.

2. Behavioral Classroom Management: Behavioral classroom management involves teaching teachers how to manage the behavior of students with ADHD in the classroom.

3. Social Skills Training: Social skills training involves teaching individuals with ADHD social skills and how to interact with others.

4. Cognitive Behavioral Therapy: Cognitive Behavioral Therapy (CBT) involves teaching individuals with ADHD how to identify and change negative thought patterns and behaviors.

Interventions

Interventions for ADHD aim to improve academic, social, and emotional functioning. Interventions include the following:

5. Academic Interventions: Academic interventions involve modifying the learning environment and teaching strategies to meet the needs of individuals with ADHD. Academic interventions may include specialized instruction, additional time for completing assignments, and use of assistive technology.

6. Behavioral Interventions: Behavioral interventions involve modifying the behavior of individuals with ADHD to improve social and emotional functioning. Behavioral interventions may include contingency management, token economy, and social skills training.

7. Parent Education: Parent education involves educating parents about ADHD and teaching them strategies to help their child manage their behavior and develop a positive relationship with their child.

8. School-Based Interventions: School-based interventions involve modifying the learning environment and teaching strategies to meet the needs of students with ADHD. School-based interventions may include behavioral classroom management and academic interventions.

Combination Therapy

Combination therapy involves the use of behavioral therapies and interventions in combination with medication. Combination therapy may be more effective than monotherapy for individuals with ADHD.

The decision to use combination therapy depends on a number of factors, including the severity of symptoms, response to treatment, and coexisting conditions. Healthcare professionals must carefully evaluate each individual and develop an individualized treatment plan.

Conclusion

In conclusion, behavioral therapies and interventions are important treatment options for individuals with ADHD. Behavioral therapies focus on changing behavior to improve social, emotional, and academic functioning. Interventions aim to improve academic, social, and emotional functioning. Combination therapy involves the use of behavioral therapies and interventions in combination with medication. The decision to use behavioral therapies and interventions depends on a number of factors and must be carefully evaluated by healthcare professionals.

Cognitive-behavioral therapy for ADHD

Attention Deficit Hyperactivity Disorder (ADHD) is a neurodevelopmental disorder that affects approximately 5-10% of school-aged children and 2-5% of adults worldwide. Cognitive-behavioral therapy (CBT) is an evidence-based intervention that has been shown to be effective in treating ADHD symptoms in both children and adults. Below we will we will explore what CBT is and how it can be used to treat ADHD.

What is Cognitive-Behavioral Therapy?

CBT is a form of psychotherapy that focuses on changing negative thought patterns and behaviors. CBT is based on the premise that negative thoughts and behaviors can be unlearned and replaced with positive ones.

CBT for ADHD involves teaching individuals with ADHD new skills and strategies to improve their attention, organization, and time management skills. CBT for ADHD also focuses on improving self-esteem and social skills.

CBT for ADHD is typically conducted in individual or group sessions and may involve homework assignments to practice new skills and strategies.

The Components of CBT for ADHD

CBT for ADHD typically includes the following components:

1. Psychoeducation: Psychoeducation involves educating individuals with ADHD and their families about ADHD and how it affects their lives.

2. Cognitive Restructuring: Cognitive restructuring involves identifying and changing negative thought patterns and replacing them with positive ones. Cognitive restructuring is used to improve self-esteem and reduce negative self-talk.

3. Behavioral Modification: Behavioral modification involves modifying negative behaviors and replacing them with positive ones. Behavioral modification is used to improve organization, time management, and social skills.

4. Problem-Solving Skills: Problem-solving skills involve identifying problems and developing strategies to solve them. Problem-solving skills are used to improve organization and time management.

5. Social Skills Training: Social skills training involves teaching individuals with ADHD how to interact with others and improve their social skills. Social skills training is used to improve relationships and reduce social isolation.

The Effectiveness of CBT for ADHD

CBT for ADHD has been shown to be effective in reducing ADHD symptoms and improving social and academic functioning in both children and adults.

A study conducted by Safren and colleagues (2010) found that CBT for ADHD was effective in improving attention, organization, and time management skills in adults with ADHD. A meta-analysis conducted by Fabiano and colleagues (2009) found that CBT for ADHD was effective in reducing ADHD symptoms and improving social and academic functioning in children with ADHD.

Conclusion

In conclusion, CBT is an evidence-based intervention that has been shown to be effective in treating ADHD symptoms in both children and adults. CBT for ADHD involves teaching individuals with ADHD new skills and strategies to improve their attention, organization, and time management skills. CBT for ADHD also focuses on improving self-esteem and social skills. CBT for ADHD is typically conducted in individual or group sessions and may involve homework assignments to practice new skills and strategies. CBT for ADHD has been shown to be effective in reducing ADHD symptoms and improving social and academic functioning.

Parent training and family therapy

Attention Deficit Hyperactivity Disorder (ADHD) is a neurodevelopmental disorder that affects many aspects of an individual's life, including their relationships with family members. Parent training and family therapy are two evidence-based interventions that can be used to help families cope with the challenges of ADHD. Below we will we will explore what parent training and family therapy are and how they can be used to help families affected by ADHD.

What is Parent Training?

Parent training involves teaching parents strategies for managing their child's behavior and developing a positive relationship with their child. Parent training for ADHD typically focuses on improving communication, providing structure and routine, and using positive reinforcement.

Parent training for ADHD may be conducted in individual or group sessions and may involve homework assignments to practice new skills and strategies.

The Components of Parent Training

Parent training for ADHD typically includes the following components:

1. Psychoeducation: Psychoeducation involves educating parents about ADHD and how it affects their child's behavior.

2. Behavioral Management: Behavioral management involves teaching parents strategies for managing their child's behavior, such as providing structure and routine, using positive reinforcement, and setting clear expectations.

3. Communication Skills: Communication skills involve teaching parents how to communicate effectively with their child and how to listen actively.

4. Problem-Solving Skills: Problem-solving skills involve teaching parents how to identify problems and develop strategies to solve them.

The Effectiveness of Parent Training for ADHD

Parent training for ADHD has been shown to be effective in improving parent-child relationships, reducing negative behaviors, and improving social and academic functioning in children with ADHD.

A study conducted by Pelham and colleagues (2014) found that parent training for ADHD was effective in reducing negative behaviors and improving social and academic functioning in children with ADHD.

What is Family Therapy?

Family therapy involves working with the entire family to improve communication, problem-solving, and relationships. Family therapy for ADHD typically focuses on improving family functioning, reducing family conflict, and improving communication.

Family therapy for ADHD may be conducted in individual or group sessions and may involve homework assignments to practice new skills and strategies.

The Components of Family Therapy

Family therapy for ADHD typically includes the following components:

5. Psychoeducation: Psychoeducation involves educating family members about ADHD and how it affects their relationships.

6. Communication Skills: Communication skills involve teaching family members how to communicate effectively with each other and how to listen actively.

7. Problem-Solving Skills: Problem-solving skills involve teaching family members how to identify problems and develop strategies to solve them.

8. Conflict Resolution: Conflict resolution involves teaching family members how to resolve conflicts in a positive and constructive manner.

The Effectiveness of Family Therapy for ADHD

Family therapy for ADHD has been shown to be effective in improving family functioning, reducing family conflict, and improving communication.

A study conducted by Cunningham and colleagues (2009) found that family therapy for ADHD was effective in improving parent-child relationships and reducing family conflict.

Conclusion

In conclusion, parent training and family therapy are two evidence-based interventions that can be used to help families cope with the challenges of ADHD. Parent training involves teaching parents strategies for managing their child's behavior and developing a positive relationship with their child. Family therapy involves working with the entire family to improve communication, problem-solving, and relationships. Both parent training and family therapy have been shown to be effective in improving family functioning, reducing family conflict, and improving social and academic functioning in children with ADHD.

Social skills training and peer interventions

Attention Deficit Hyperactivity Disorder (ADHD) is a neurodevelopmental disorder that can impact an individual's social skills and ability to interact with peers. Social skills training and peer interventions are two evidence-based interventions that can be used to improve social skills and relationships with peers for individuals with ADHD. Below we will we will explore what social skills training and peer interventions are and how they can be used to help individuals with ADHD.

What is Social Skills Training?

Social skills training involves teaching individuals with ADHD new skills and strategies to improve their social skills and ability to interact with peers. Social skills training for ADHD typically focuses on improving communication, social problem-solving, and self-esteem.

Social skills training for ADHD may be conducted in individual or group sessions and may involve homework assignments to practice new skills and strategies.

The Components of Social Skills Training

Social skills training for ADHD typically includes the following components:

1. Psychoeducation: Psychoeducation involves educating individuals with ADHD about their disorder and how it affects their social skills.

2. Communication Skills: Communication skills involve teaching individuals with ADHD how to communicate effectively with peers and how to listen actively.

3. Problem-Solving Skills: Problem-solving skills involve teaching individuals with ADHD how to identify social problems and develop strategies to solve them.

4. Self-Esteem Building: Self-esteem building involves teaching individuals with ADHD how to develop a positive self-image and improve their self-confidence.

The Effectiveness of Social Skills Training for ADHD

Social skills training for ADHD has been shown to be effective in improving social skills, reducing social isolation, and improving social and academic functioning.

A study conducted by Mautone and colleagues (2012) found that social skills training for ADHD was effective in improving social skills and reducing social isolation in children with ADHD.

What are Peer Interventions?

Peer interventions involve working with peers to improve social skills and relationships. Peer interventions for ADHD typically involve pairing individuals with ADHD with peers who have similar interests and hobbies.

Peer interventions for ADHD may involve a structured program, such as a social skills group, or may involve informal interactions between peers.

The Components of Peer Interventions

Peer interventions for ADHD typically include the following components:

5. Psychoeducation: Psychoeducation involves educating peers about ADHD and how it affects their friend.

6. Social Skills Training: Social skills training involves teaching peers how to interact with their friend with ADHD and how to communicate effectively.

7. Support and Encouragement: Support and encouragement involves providing positive feedback to the individual with ADHD and helping them to feel included and accepted.

The Effectiveness of Peer Interventions for ADHD

Peer interventions for ADHD have been shown to be effective in improving social skills, reducing social isolation, and improving social and academic functioning.

A study conducted by Hoza and colleagues (2005) found that a structured peer intervention program was effective in improving social skills and reducing social isolation in children with ADHD.

Conclusion

In conclusion, social skills training and peer interventions are two evidence-based interventions that can be used to improve social skills and relationships with peers for individuals with ADHD. Social skills training involves teaching individuals with ADHD new skills and strategies to improve their social skills and ability to interact with peers. Peer interventions involve working with peers to improve social skills and relationships. Both social skills training and peer interventions have been shown to be effective in improving social skills, reducing social isolation, and improving social and academic functioning in individuals with ADHD.

Chapter Six

ADHD Coaching and Support

Attention Deficit Hyperactivity Disorder (ADHD) is a neurodevelopmental disorder that can impact an individual's ability to manage tasks and stay organized. ADHD coaching and support are two evidence-based interventions that can be used to help individuals with ADHD develop coping skills and strategies to manage their symptoms. Below we will we will explore what ADHD coaching and support are and how they can be used to help individuals with ADHD.

What is ADHD Coaching?

ADHD coaching involves working with a coach to develop coping skills and strategies to manage symptoms of ADHD. ADHD coaches typically work with individuals with ADHD to identify areas of difficulty and develop a plan to improve their functioning.

ADHD coaching may be conducted in individual or group sessions and may involve homework assignments to practice new skills and strategies.

The Components of ADHD Coaching

ADHD coaching typically includes the following components:

1. Goal-Setting: Goal-setting involves working with the individual with ADHD to identify areas of difficulty and develop goals to improve their functioning.

2. Skill-Building: Skill-building involves teaching individuals with ADHD new coping skills and strategies to manage their symptoms.

3. Accountability: Accountability involves setting up a system of accountability to ensure that the individual with ADHD is practicing new skills and strategies.

4. Support: Support involves providing emotional support and encouragement to the individual with ADHD.

The Effectiveness of ADHD Coaching

ADHD coaching has been shown to be effective in improving executive functioning, reducing symptoms of ADHD, and improving overall functioning.

A study conducted by Safren and colleagues (2010) found that ADHD coaching was effective in improving executive functioning and reducing symptoms of ADHD in adults with ADHD.

What is ADHD Support?

ADHD support involves working with a support group or mental health professional to manage the challenges of ADHD. ADHD support may involve education about ADHD, as well as emotional support and encouragement.

ADHD support may be provided in individual or group sessions and may involve homework assignments to practice new skills and strategies.

The Components of ADHD Support

ADHD support typically includes the following components:

5. Psychoeducation: Psychoeducation involves educating individuals with ADHD about their disorder and how it affects their functioning.

6. Emotional Support: Emotional support involves providing individuals with ADHD with a safe and supportive environment to discuss their challenges and concerns.

7. Encouragement: Encouragement involves providing positive feedback and encouragement to individuals with ADHD.

The Effectiveness of ADHD Support

ADHD support has been shown to be effective in improving emotional well-being, reducing stress, and improving overall functioning.

A study conducted by Chronis-Tuscano and colleagues (2010) found that group-based support for parents of children with ADHD was effective in reducing parenting stress and improving emotional well-being.

Conclusion

In conclusion, ADHD coaching and support are two evidence-based interventions that can be used to help individuals with ADHD develop coping skills and strategies to manage their symptoms. ADHD coaching involves working with a coach to develop coping skills and strategies to manage symptoms of ADHD, while ADHD support involves working with a support group or mental health professional to manage the challenges of ADHD. Both ADHD coaching and support have been shown to be effective in improving functioning and reducing symptoms of ADHD.

The role of ADHD coaches in management and support

Attention Deficit Hyperactivity Disorder (ADHD) is a neurodevelopmental disorder that can impact an individual's ability to manage tasks and stay organized. ADHD coaches play an important role in the management and support of individuals with ADHD. Below we will we will explore what ADHD coaches are, what their role is in managing and supporting individuals with ADHD, and how they can be beneficial to individuals with ADHD.

What is an ADHD Coach?

An ADHD coach is a trained professional who works with individuals with ADHD to develop coping skills and strategies to manage their symptoms. ADHD coaches are typically trained in coaching techniques, as well as in the specific challenges associated with ADHD.

ADHD coaches may work in a variety of settings, including private practice, schools, and clinics. They may work with individuals of all ages, including children, adolescents, and adults.

What is the Role of an ADHD Coach?

The role of an ADHD coach is to help individuals with ADHD develop coping skills and strategies to manage their symptoms. ADHD coaches work with individuals with ADHD to identify areas of difficulty and develop a plan to improve their functioning.

The role of an ADHD coach may include the following:

1. Goal-Setting: ADHD coaches work with individuals with ADHD to set specific, measurable goals that are achievable.

2. Skill-Building: ADHD coaches teach individuals with ADHD new coping skills and strategies to manage their symptoms.

3. Accountability: ADHD coaches hold individuals with ADHD accountable for practicing new skills and strategies.

4. Support: ADHD coaches provide emotional support and encouragement to individuals with ADHD.

5. Advocacy: ADHD coaches may advocate for individuals with ADHD in school or work settings.

The Benefits of ADHD Coaching

ADHD coaching has been shown to be effective in improving executive functioning, reducing symptoms of ADHD, and improving overall functioning.

A study conducted by Safren and colleagues (2010) found that ADHD coaching was effective in improving executive functioning and reducing symptoms of ADHD in adults with ADHD.

Another study conducted by Weiss and colleagues (2008) found that ADHD coaching was effective in improving academic and organizational skills in college students with ADHD.

ADHD coaching can also be beneficial for children with ADHD. A study conducted by Gray and colleagues (2012) found that ADHD coaching was effective in improving homework completion and reducing parent-child conflict in children with ADHD.

Conclusion

In conclusion, ADHD coaches play an important role in the management and support of individuals with ADHD. ADHD coaches work with individuals with ADHD to develop coping skills and strategies to manage their symptoms. The role of an ADHD coach may include goal-setting, skill-building, accountability, support, and advocacy. ADHD coaching has been shown to be effective in improving executive functioning, reducing symptoms of ADHD, and improving overall functioning. ADHD coaching can be beneficial for individuals of all ages, including children, adolescents, and adults.

Strategies for selecting an ADHD coach

Selecting the right ADHD coach is an important step in managing symptoms of Attention Deficit Hyperactivity Disorder (ADHD). An ADHD coach can help individuals with ADHD develop coping skills and strategies to manage their symptoms, and provide support and encouragement. Below we will we will explore strategies for selecting an ADHD coach, including the qualities to look for and questions to ask.

Qualities to Look for in an ADHD Coach

When selecting an ADHD coach, there are several qualities to look for:

1. Training and Credentials: Look for an ADHD coach who has received specialized training in coaching techniques and the specific challenges associated with ADHD. It is also important to look for an ADHD coach who has appropriate credentials and is licensed or certified.

2. Experience: Look for an ADHD coach who has experience working with individuals with ADHD. An experienced ADHD coach will have a better understanding of the challenges associated with ADHD and will be better equipped to provide effective coaching.

3. Empathy and Compassion: Look for an ADHD coach who is empathetic and compassionate. An ADHD coach who is able to understand and relate to the challenges faced by individuals with ADHD can provide more effective coaching.

4. Flexibility: Look for an ADHD coach who is flexible and able to adapt to the needs of the individual. Individuals with ADHD may have different

needs and preferences, and a coach who is able to adapt to these needs can provide more effective coaching.

Questions to Ask When Selecting an ADHD Coach

When selecting an ADHD coach, it is important to ask questions to ensure that the coach is the right fit for you. Some questions to ask include:

What is your experience working with individuals with ADHD?

What is your training and credentials?

What coaching techniques do you use?

What is your approach to coaching?

What is your availability?

How do you track progress?

What is your policy on confidentiality?

What is your policy on cancellations?

What is your fee structure?

Do you provide a free consultation or trial session?

Conclusion

In conclusion, selecting the right ADHD coach is an important step in managing symptoms of ADHD. When selecting an ADHD coach, it is important to look for an ADHD coach who has specialized training and credentials, experience working with individuals with ADHD, empathy and compassion, and flexibility. It is also important to ask questions to ensure that the coach is the right fit for you. By selecting the right ADHD coach, individuals with ADHD can develop coping skills and strategies to manage their symptoms and improve their overall functioning.

Benefits of support groups and networks

Living with Attention Deficit Hyperactivity Disorder (ADHD) can be challenging, but joining a support group or network can offer many benefits. Support groups and networks provide individuals with ADHD with the opportunity to connect with others who share similar experiences and challenges. Below we will we will explore the benefits of support groups and networks for individuals with ADHD.

Benefits of Support Groups and Networks

1. Emotional Support: Joining a support group or network can provide individuals with ADHD with emotional support. Individuals with ADHD may feel isolated and alone, but joining a support group or network can help them feel less alone and provide a sense of community.

2. Shared Experiences: Support groups and networks provide individuals with ADHD with the opportunity to share their experiences with others who have similar challenges. This can be validating and reassuring, as individuals with ADHD often struggle to feel understood.

3. Coping Strategies: Support groups and networks can provide individuals with ADHD with coping strategies and techniques to manage their symptoms. Individuals with ADHD can learn from others who have developed effective coping strategies, which can be helpful in improving their overall functioning.

4. Education: Support groups and networks can provide individuals with ADHD with education about the disorder and its management. This can

help individuals with ADHD better understand their condition and make informed decisions about treatment options.

5. Reduced Stigma: Joining a support group or network can help reduce the stigma associated with ADHD. Individuals with ADHD may feel judged or misunderstood by others, but being part of a group of individuals who share similar experiences can help reduce feelings of stigma.

6. Accountability: Support groups and networks can provide individuals with ADHD with a sense of accountability. By sharing their experiences and progress with others in the group, individuals with ADHD may feel more motivated to stick to their goals and commitments.

7. Networking: Support groups and networks can provide individuals with ADHD with networking opportunities. Individuals with ADHD may meet others who can offer support and advice in areas such as education, career, and parenting.

Conclusion

In conclusion, joining a support group or network can provide individuals with ADHD with many benefits, including emotional support, shared experiences, coping strategies, education, reduced stigma, accountability, and networking opportunities. It is important for individuals with ADHD to seek out support and connect with others who share similar experiences and challenges. Support groups and networks can be a valuable resource for individuals with ADHD as they navigate their journey of managing their symptoms and improving their overall functioning.

Chapter Seven

Nutrition and Lifestyle Factors

Attention Deficit Hyperactivity Disorder (ADHD) is a neurodevelopmental disorder that can impact an individual's ability to focus and manage tasks. While medication and therapy can be effective in managing symptoms, nutrition and lifestyle factors can also play an important role. Below we will we will explore the impact of nutrition and lifestyle factors on ADHD and strategies for improving them.

Nutrition Factors

1. Omega-3 Fatty Acids: Omega-3 fatty acids are essential fats that are important for brain function. Research has shown that omega-3 supplements may improve symptoms of ADHD, particularly in children.

2. Protein: Protein is important for brain function and can help stabilize blood sugar levels. Eating protein-rich foods such as eggs, chicken, and nuts can help individuals with ADHD maintain focus and concentration.

3. Complex Carbohydrates: Complex carbohydrates, such as whole grains, can provide sustained energy and help stabilize blood sugar levels. This can be particularly helpful for individuals with ADHD, who may struggle with impulsivity and hyperactivity.

4. Vitamins and Minerals: Adequate intake of vitamins and minerals, such as iron, zinc, and vitamin D, can be important for brain function. Individuals with ADHD may benefit from taking supplements or increasing their intake of foods rich in these nutrients.

Lifestyle Factors

5. Exercise: Exercise can be an effective strategy for managing symptoms of ADHD. Exercise releases endorphins, which can improve mood and help individuals with ADHD focus and concentrate.

6. Sleep: Adequate sleep is important for brain function and can help individuals with ADHD manage symptoms such as impulsivity and hyperactivity. Establishing a regular sleep routine and avoiding caffeine and electronic devices before bed can help improve sleep quality.

7. Stress Management: Stress can exacerbate symptoms of ADHD. Developing strategies for managing stress, such as mindfulness meditation or deep breathing exercises, can help individuals with ADHD manage their symptoms.

8. Organization: Individuals with ADHD may struggle with organization and time management. Developing strategies for organizing tasks and keeping a schedule can help individuals with ADHD stay on track and manage their symptoms.

In conclusion, nutrition and lifestyle factors can play an important role in managing symptoms of ADHD. Adequate intake of omega-3 fatty acids, protein, complex carbohydrates, vitamins, and minerals can be important for brain function. Exercise, adequate sleep, stress management, and organization can also be effective strategies for managing symptoms of ADHD. By incorporating these strategies into their daily routine, individuals with ADHD can improve their overall functioning and manage their symptoms more effectively.

The impact of diet and nutrition on ADHD symptoms

Attention Deficit Hyperactivity Disorder (ADHD) is a neurodevelopmental disorder characterized by symptoms such as hyperactivity, impulsivity, and difficulty with attention and focus. While medication and therapy can be effective in managing ADHD symptoms, recent research has also shown that diet and nutrition may play a role. Below we will we will explore the impact of diet and nutrition on ADHD symptoms.

Impact of Diet on ADHD Symptoms

1. Sugar: Sugar has long been thought to exacerbate symptoms of ADHD, but recent research has shown mixed results. Some studies suggest that sugar intake may worsen hyperactivity and impulsivity, while others have found no significant link between sugar and ADHD symptoms.

2. Food Additives: Some food additives, such as artificial colors and preservatives, have been linked to worsening of ADHD symptoms. The mechanism for this is not fully understood, but some studies suggest that certain food additives may interfere with brain function.

3. Caffeine: Caffeine is a stimulant that can improve attention and focus in some individuals, but may worsen symptoms of hyperactivity and impulsivity in others.

4. Omega-3 Fatty Acids: Omega-3 fatty acids are essential fats that are important for brain function. Research has shown that omega-3 supplements may improve symptoms of ADHD, particularly in children.

5. Protein: Protein is important for brain function and can help stabilize blood sugar levels. Eating protein-rich foods such as eggs, chicken, and nuts can help individuals with ADHD maintain focus and concentration.

Impact of Nutrition on ADHD Symptoms

6. Iron: Iron is important for brain function and deficiency may be linked to ADHD symptoms. Individuals with ADHD may benefit from increasing their intake of iron-rich foods such as red meat, poultry, and beans.

7. Zinc: Zinc is important for brain function and deficiency may be linked to ADHD symptoms. Individuals with ADHD may benefit from increasing their intake of zinc-rich foods such as oysters, beef, and fortified cereals.

8. Vitamin D: Adequate intake of vitamin D is important for brain function. Individuals with ADHD may benefit from increasing their intake of vitamin D-rich foods such as fatty fish, fortified dairy products, and egg yolks.

9. Magnesium: Magnesium is important for brain function and deficiency may be linked to ADHD symptoms. Individuals with ADHD may benefit from increasing their intake of magnesium-rich foods such as almonds, spinach, and dark chocolate.

Conclusion

In conclusion, diet and nutrition may play a role in managing symptoms of ADHD. While the impact of sugar and food additives on ADHD symptoms is still unclear, omega-3 fatty acids, protein, iron, zinc, vitamin D, and magnesium have all been shown to be important for brain function and may help improve symptoms of ADHD. Individuals with ADHD may benefit from working with a healthcare professional or registered dietitian to develop a nutrition plan that meets their individual needs and supports optimal brain function.

Exercise, sleep, and other lifestyle factors

Attention Deficit Hyperactivity Disorder (ADHD) is a neurodevelopmental disorder that can impact an individual's ability to focus, organize, and manage tasks. While medication and therapy can be effective in managing symptoms, lifestyle factors such as exercise, sleep, and stress management can also play an important role. Below we will we will explore the impact of exercise, sleep, and other lifestyle factors on ADHD and strategies for improving them.

Exercise

Exercise is a powerful tool for managing symptoms of ADHD. Physical activity releases endorphins, which can improve mood and help individuals with ADHD focus and concentrate. Studies have shown that exercise can improve attention, reduce hyperactivity, and improve impulse control in individuals with ADHD. Exercise also promotes brain health and may help individuals with ADHD develop better cognitive control. Strategies for incorporating exercise into daily routine can include walking, cycling, swimming, or participating in sports.

Sleep

Adequate sleep is important for brain function and can help individuals with ADHD manage symptoms such as impulsivity and hyperactivity. Studies have shown that individuals with ADHD may be more prone to sleep disturbances, including difficulty falling asleep and staying asleep. Establishing a regular sleep routine and avoiding caffeine and electronic devices before bed can help improve sleep quality. Strategies for improving sleep can also include creating a relaxing sleep environment, such as keeping the bedroom cool and dark, and practicing relaxation techniques such as deep breathing or meditation.

Stress Management

Stress can exacerbate symptoms of ADHD. Developing strategies for managing stress, such as mindfulness meditation or deep breathing exercises, can help individuals with ADHD manage their symptoms. Other stress-management strategies may include regular exercise, social support, and time-management skills.

Organization

Individuals with ADHD may struggle with organization and time management. Developing strategies for organizing tasks and keeping a schedule can help individuals with ADHD stay on track and manage their symptoms. Strategies may include using a planner or scheduling app, breaking tasks into smaller, more manageable steps, and setting reminders or alarms to stay on schedule.

Diet and Nutrition

As discussed in a separate chapter, diet and nutrition can also play an important role in managing symptoms of ADHD. Adequate intake of omega-3 fatty acids, protein, complex carbohydrates, vitamins, and minerals can be important for brain function. Individuals with ADHD may benefit from working with a healthcare professional or registered dietitian to develop a nutrition plan that meets their individual needs and supports optimal brain function.

Conclusion

In conclusion, lifestyle factors such as exercise, sleep, stress management, organization, and diet and nutrition can all play an important role in managing symptoms of ADHD. Incorporating regular exercise, establishing a regular sleep routine, developing stress-management strategies, organizing tasks and keeping a schedule, and following a nutritious diet can all help individuals with ADHD manage their symptoms more effectively.

By incorporating these strategies into their daily routine, individuals with ADHD can improve their overall functioning and quality of life.

Strategies for implementing healthy habits

Individuals with Attention Deficit Hyperactivity Disorder (ADHD) often struggle with maintaining healthy habits, such as exercise, sleep, and nutrition. However, developing and implementing healthy habits can be an effective strategy for managing symptoms of ADHD. Below we will we will explore strategies for implementing healthy habits that can benefit individuals with ADHD.

1. Create a routine: Establishing a consistent routine can be beneficial for individuals with ADHD. This can include setting regular meal times, exercise times, and sleep schedules. Having a routine can help with time management and organization, two areas that individuals with ADHD often struggle with.

2. Set achievable goals: Setting achievable goals can help individuals with ADHD feel a sense of accomplishment and improve motivation. When setting goals, it is important to be realistic and break them down into smaller, more manageable tasks. This can help prevent feeling overwhelmed and discouraged.

3. Use reminders: Individuals with ADHD may struggle with forgetfulness and impulsivity. Using reminders, such as alarms on a phone or a daily planner, can be helpful in staying on track with healthy habits. Reminders can be used for tasks such as taking medication, drinking water, or going for a walk.

4. Seek support: Seeking support from friends, family, or a healthcare professional can be beneficial in developing and maintaining healthy habits.

A support system can provide encouragement, accountability, and helpful tips for managing symptoms of ADHD.

5. Focus on strengths: Individuals with ADHD often have unique strengths, such as creativity and problem-solving skills. Focusing on these strengths can help boost confidence and motivation. For example, individuals with ADHD may excel in activities such as music or art, which can be incorporated into a healthy lifestyle.

6. Use positive self-talk: Negative self-talk can be detrimental to maintaining healthy habits. Using positive self-talk, such as "I can do this" or "I am making progress", can help improve self-esteem and motivation.

7. Make it enjoyable: Healthy habits do not have to be boring or tedious. Finding enjoyable activities, such as dancing, hiking, or cooking, can make healthy habits more sustainable and enjoyable.

8. Track progress: Tracking progress can help individuals with ADHD stay motivated and see improvements over time. This can be done through a journal, a habit tracker app, or by setting specific milestones to work towards.

In conclusion, implementing healthy habits can be a powerful strategy for managing symptoms of ADHD. Creating a routine, setting achievable goals, using reminders, seeking support, focusing on strengths, using positive self-talk, making it enjoyable, and tracking progress are all effective strategies for implementing healthy habits. By incorporating these strategies into their daily routine, individuals with ADHD can improve their overall functioning and quality of life.

Chapter Eight

ADHD and Education

Attention Deficit Hyperactivity Disorder (ADHD) can impact an individual's ability to learn and succeed in an educational setting. However, with appropriate accommodations and support, individuals with ADHD can thrive in their academic pursuits. Below we will we will explore the impact of ADHD on education and strategies for supporting academic success.

Impact of ADHD on Education

Individuals with ADHD may experience difficulty with attention, organization, and impulse control, all of which can impact their ability to learn in a classroom setting. They may struggle with completing assignments on time, following directions, and staying focused during lectures or discussions. These difficulties can lead to academic challenges, such as lower grades, incomplete assignments, and disciplinary issues.

Accommodations and Strategies for Academic Success

Accommodations and strategies can be implemented to support individuals with ADHD in their academic pursuits. Some effective accommodations and strategies include:

1. Classroom modifications: Teachers can make modifications in the classroom, such as seating the student near the front of the room, minimizing distractions, and breaking down complex assignments into smaller, more manageable tasks.

2. Accommodations for testing: Accommodations such as extended time, breaks, and alternative testing methods, such as oral exams, can help students with ADHD perform to their full potential on exams.

3. Use of technology: Technology, such as text-to-speech software and digital organizers, can help students with ADHD stay organized and focused.

4. Behavioral interventions: Behavioral interventions, such as token economies or positive reinforcement, can help encourage and reward positive behavior.

5. Medication: Medication can be an effective tool for managing symptoms of ADHD and improving academic performance. However, medication should only be used under the supervision of a healthcare professional.

6. Study skills training: Learning effective study skills, such as time management and note-taking strategies, can help individuals with ADHD stay focused and organized.

7. Parent and teacher collaboration: Collaboration between parents and teachers can be key in ensuring the success of a student with ADHD. Regular communication can help identify challenges and strategies for success.

In conclusion, ADHD can present unique challenges in an educational setting, but appropriate accommodations and support can help individuals with ADHD succeed academically. Classroom modifications, accommodations for testing, use of technology, behavioral interventions, medication, study skills training, and parent and teacher collaboration are all effective strategies for supporting academic success. By implementing these strategies, individuals with ADHD can reach their full potential and achieve academic success.

Classroom accommodations and supports for students with ADHD

Attention Deficit Hyperactivity Disorder (ADHD) can impact a student's ability to succeed in a classroom setting. However, with appropriate accommodations and supports, students with ADHD can thrive academically. Below we will we will explore some effective classroom accommodations and supports for students with ADHD.

1. Preferential seating: Students with ADHD may benefit from sitting in a specific area of the classroom to minimize distractions and help them focus on the teacher. Sitting in the front of the room or away from distractions such as windows or doors can be beneficial.

2. Visual aids: Visual aids such as graphic organizers or visual schedules can help students with ADHD stay organized and on task. These aids can help break down tasks into smaller, more manageable steps, making it easier for students to follow through on assignments.

3. Shortened assignments: Students with ADHD may become overwhelmed with lengthy assignments. Shortened assignments can help students manage their time and stay focused on the task at hand.

4. Extended time on assignments: Students with ADHD may require more time to complete assignments due to difficulties with attention and organization. Providing extended time can give students with ADHD the opportunity to complete assignments at their own pace and reduce feelings of stress and anxiety.

5. Fidget tools: Providing fidget tools such as stress balls or fidget spinners can help students with ADHD stay focused and reduce impulsivity by providing a physical outlet for energy.

6. Breaks: Frequent breaks can help students with ADHD manage their energy levels and reduce feelings of restlessness. Short breaks to stretch, move, or take a quick walk can be beneficial.

7. Positive reinforcement: Providing positive feedback and praise can help students with ADHD feel motivated and encouraged to continue working hard. Rewarding good behavior can also help reinforce positive habits and improve academic performance.

8. Verbal cues: Providing verbal cues or reminders can help students with ADHD stay on task and reduce impulsivity. Cues such as "pay attention" or "stay on task" can help students stay focused and engaged in the lesson.

9. Checklists: Providing checklists for assignments and tasks can help students with ADHD stay organized and reduce forgetfulness. Checklists can also provide a sense of accomplishment as students complete each item on the list.

10. Collaboration with parents: Collaboration with parents can be key in ensuring the success of a student with ADHD. Regular communication can help identify challenges and strategies for success.

In conclusion, providing classroom accommodations and supports can help students with ADHD succeed academically. Preferential seating, visual aids, shortened assignments, extended time on assignments, fidget tools, breaks, positive reinforcement, verbal cues, checklists, and collaboration with parents are all effective strategies for supporting students with ADHD in the classroom. By implementing these strategies, students with ADHD can reach their full potential and achieve academic success.

Working with teachers and school staff

Working with teachers and school staff is an essential part of supporting students with Attention Deficit Hyperactivity Disorder (ADHD) in the classroom. By working together, teachers and school staff can create a supportive and effective learning environment that meets the unique needs of students with ADHD. Below we will we will explore strategies for working with teachers and school staff to support students with ADHD.

1. Communicate with teachers: Communication with teachers is essential in ensuring that students with ADHD are receiving the appropriate support and accommodations in the classroom. Parents and caregivers should communicate regularly with teachers to discuss the student's progress, any challenges they may be facing, and any strategies that have been effective in managing their symptoms.

2. Create an individualized education plan (IEP): An IEP is a legal document that outlines the specific accommodations and supports that a student with ADHD requires to succeed academically. The IEP should be developed in collaboration with parents, teachers, and school staff to ensure that it addresses the student's unique needs and challenges.

3. Provide training for teachers: Providing training for teachers on ADHD can help them better understand the condition and how it impacts their students. Training can also provide teachers with effective strategies for managing students with ADHD in the classroom.

4. Develop a behavior plan: A behavior plan can help students with ADHD understand what is expected of them in the classroom and provide them with clear expectations for their behavior. The behavior plan should outline the consequences of inappropriate behavior and provide positive reinforcement for good behavior.

5. Use assistive technology: Assistive technology, such as text-to-speech software or digital organizers, can help students with ADHD stay orga-

nized and focused in the classroom. Teachers and school staff should be trained in the use of these tools and should incorporate them into the student's learning plan as appropriate.

6. Develop a system for communication: A system for communication between teachers, school staff, and parents can help ensure that everyone is on the same page and working towards the same goals for the student with ADHD. This may include regular progress reports, meetings, or other forms of communication.

7. Provide social-emotional support: Students with ADHD may require additional social-emotional support to succeed in the classroom. Teachers and school staff should be trained in techniques for providing emotional support, such as mindfulness exercises or counseling.

8. Encourage physical activity: Physical activity can be an effective way to manage symptoms of ADHD. Teachers and school staff should encourage physical activity, such as recess or movement breaks, to help students with ADHD manage their energy levels and stay focused in the classroom.

In conclusion, working with teachers and school staff is essential in supporting students with ADHD in the classroom. By communicating regularly, developing an individualized education plan, providing training for teachers, developing a behavior plan, using assistive technology, developing a system for communication, providing social-emotional support, and encouraging physical activity, teachers and school staff can create a supportive and effective learning environment for students with ADHD.

Navigating the special education process

Navigating the special education process can be a challenging and overwhelming task for parents and caregivers of students with Attention

Deficit Hyperactivity Disorder (ADHD). However, it is essential to understand the special education process and the rights of students with disabilities to ensure they receive the appropriate support and accommodations to succeed academically. Below we will we will explore strategies for navigating the special education process for students with ADHD.

1. Understand the laws: The Individuals with Disabilities Education Act (IDEA) is a federal law that requires schools to provide appropriate education and services for students with disabilities. IDEA also requires schools to develop an Individualized Education Plan (IEP) for students with disabilities, including students with ADHD. It is essential to understand the laws to ensure that your child's rights are being protected.

2. Identify the need for special education: Parents and caregivers should work with teachers and school staff to determine if a student requires special education services. A student with ADHD may require special education services if their symptoms significantly impact their ability to learn and succeed in the classroom.

3. Request an evaluation: If it is determined that a student requires special education services, parents and caregivers should request an evaluation from the school. The evaluation will assess the student's academic performance, behavior, and any other factors that may impact their ability to learn.

4. Participate in the evaluation process: Parents and caregivers should participate in the evaluation process by providing information about the student's medical history, behavior, and academic performance. It is essential to be as thorough as possible in providing information to ensure that the evaluation accurately reflects the student's needs.

5. Review and sign the IEP: Once the evaluation is complete, the school will develop an Individualized Education Plan (IEP) for the student. The

IEP outlines the specific accommodations and support the student requires to succeed academically. Parents and caregivers should review and sign the IEP to ensure that it addresses the student's unique needs and challenges.

6. Participate in the IEP meeting: Parents and caregivers should participate in the IEP meeting to ensure that the IEP addresses the student's needs and provides appropriate accommodations and support. During the meeting, parents and caregivers should ask questions and provide input to ensure that the IEP is tailored to the student's needs.

7. Monitor progress: It is essential to monitor the student's progress regularly to ensure that the IEP is effective and that the student is making progress academically. Parents and caregivers should request regular progress reports and should communicate regularly with teachers and school staff to ensure that the student's needs are being met.

In conclusion, navigating the special education process can be a daunting task for parents and caregivers of students with ADHD. However, it is essential to understand the laws and the rights of students with disabilities to ensure that they receive the appropriate support and accommodations to succeed academically. By identifying the need for special education, requesting an evaluation, participating in the evaluation process, reviewing and signing the IEP, participating in the IEP meeting, and monitoring progress, parents and caregivers can navigate the special education process effectively and ensure that their child's needs are being met.

Chapter Nine

College and ADHD

Going to college can be an exciting and challenging experience for any student. However, for students with Attention Deficit Hyperactivity Disorder (ADHD), the college experience can be particularly challenging. The transition to college can be overwhelming, and students with ADHD may struggle to manage their time, stay organized, and keep up with their academic workload. Below we will we will explore strategies for college students with ADHD to succeed academically.

1. Self-advocacy: Students with ADHD should learn how to advocate for themselves in the college setting. They should communicate with professors and disability service providers to ensure that they receive the appropriate accommodations and support. Self-advocacy also involves learning how to manage their ADHD symptoms effectively.

2. Develop time management skills: Time management is critical for college students with ADHD. Students should learn how to prioritize tasks, break down assignments into manageable tasks, and create a schedule that allows for adequate time for studying and completing assignments. Time management apps and tools can be helpful for students with ADHD.

3. Create a study-friendly environment: Creating a study-friendly environment can be helpful for students with ADHD. This can involve finding a quiet and organized space to study, removing distractions such as social media and television, and using tools such as noise-canceling headphones.

4. Seek out academic support: Many colleges offer academic support services such as tutoring, writing centers, and study groups. Students with ADHD should take advantage of these services to stay on top of their academic workload and improve their academic performance.

5. Develop healthy habits: Developing healthy habits such as getting adequate sleep, exercising regularly, and eating a healthy diet can help students with ADHD manage their symptoms effectively. Students should also avoid substance abuse as it can worsen ADHD symptoms.

6. Join a support group: Joining a support group can be helpful for college students with ADHD. Support groups provide a safe and supportive environment for students to share their experiences and learn from others who are going through similar challenges.

7. Stay organized: Staying organized is critical for college students with ADHD. Students should use tools such as planners and calendars to keep track of their assignments and deadlines. They should also keep their living space and study area organized to avoid distractions and reduce stress.

In conclusion, college can be a challenging experience for students with ADHD. However, by developing self-advocacy skills, time management skills, creating a study-friendly environment, seeking out academic support, developing healthy habits, joining a support group, and staying organized, students with ADHD can succeed academically in college. It is essential for students with ADHD to communicate with professors and disability service providers to ensure that they receive the appropriate accommodations and support to help them succeed academically.

Preparing for college with ADHD

Preparing for college can be a challenging experience for any student, but for those with Attention Deficit Hyperactivity Disorder (ADHD), the transition can be particularly overwhelming. However, with proper preparation, students with ADHD can have a successful and fulfilling college experience. Below we will we will explore strategies for preparing for college with ADHD.

1. Start planning early: It is essential to start planning for college early, preferably in the junior year of high school. Students should begin researching colleges, exploring their interests and strengths, and identifying potential majors. It is also essential to research colleges that offer support services for students with ADHD.

2. Seek support: Students with ADHD should seek support from their high school guidance counselor, parents, and healthcare providers. Guidance counselors can help students identify colleges that offer support services for students with ADHD, while healthcare providers can help students manage their symptoms and develop coping strategies.

3. Visit colleges: Visiting colleges can help students with ADHD get a better sense of what college life is like and what support services are available. It is also an opportunity to meet with disability service providers to learn about the accommodations that are available to students with ADHD.

4. Develop study skills: Developing study skills is essential for success in college, particularly for students with ADHD. High school students with ADHD should learn effective study strategies such as breaking down assignments into smaller tasks, using visual aids, and finding a quiet study space. These skills can be applied in college to help students manage their workload effectively.

5. Learn time management skills: Time management is critical for success in college. Students with ADHD should learn how to prioritize tasks,

create a schedule, and avoid procrastination. Time management apps and tools can be helpful for students with ADHD.

6. Develop healthy habits: Developing healthy habits such as getting adequate sleep, exercising regularly, and eating a healthy diet can help students with ADHD manage their symptoms effectively. Students should also avoid substance abuse as it can worsen ADHD symptoms.

7. Consider taking a gap year: Taking a gap year can be an option for students with ADHD who need extra time to develop skills and strategies to manage their symptoms effectively. During a gap year, students can focus on developing study skills, time management skills, and healthy habits.

8. Communicate with professors: Communication with professors is critical for students with ADHD. Students should communicate their needs and accommodations to professors early in the semester. They should also seek out help from professors if they are struggling with the coursework.

In conclusion, preparing for college with ADHD requires careful planning and support. By starting early, seeking support, visiting colleges, developing study skills, learning time management skills, developing healthy habits, considering taking a gap year, and communicating with professors, students with ADHD can have a successful and fulfilling college experience. It is essential to research colleges that offer support services for students with ADHD and to seek out guidance from healthcare providers and guidance counselors. With proper preparation and support, students with ADHD can thrive in college and achieve their academic goals.

Accommodations and support services in higher education

As more and more students with disabilities pursue higher education, colleges and universities are increasingly offering accommodations and support services to meet their needs. This is particularly important for students with Attention Deficit Hyperactivity Disorder (ADHD), who may require specific accommodations to succeed in college. Below we will we will explore some of the accommodations and support services available to students with ADHD in higher education.

1. Disability Services: Most colleges and universities have an office of disability services that offers accommodations and support services for students with disabilities, including ADHD. Disability services can provide a range of accommodations, such as extended time on tests, note-taking services, priority registration, and assistive technology.

2. Academic Coaching: Academic coaching is a one-on-one service that helps students with ADHD develop study skills, time management skills, and organizational strategies. Academic coaches can help students identify their strengths and weaknesses and develop personalized plans for success in college.

3. Counseling Services: Counseling services can provide support for students with ADHD who are struggling with anxiety, depression, or other mental health issues. Counselors can help students manage stress, develop coping strategies, and maintain a healthy work-life balance.

4. Study Groups: Study groups can be an effective way for students with ADHD to learn course material and develop study skills. Working with peers can help students stay focused and engaged, and can provide a sense of community and support.

5. Assistive Technology: Assistive technology, such as speech-to-text software, can be a helpful tool for students with ADHD who struggle with writing and typing. Other assistive technology, such as noise-cancelling

headphones or fidget toys, can help students with ADHD stay focused and engaged during class.

6. Peer Mentoring: Peer mentoring programs can connect students with ADHD to other students who have successfully navigated college with ADHD. Peer mentors can offer advice, support, and guidance to help students with ADHD succeed in college.

7. Support Groups: Support groups can provide a sense of community and support for students with ADHD. Students can share their experiences, offer advice, and provide encouragement to one another. Support groups can be offered by the college or university, or students can seek out support groups in their community.

8. Flexibility with Attendance and Deadlines: Students with ADHD may require flexibility with attendance and deadlines due to their symptoms. Colleges and universities can offer flexible attendance policies and extensions on deadlines to accommodate students with ADHD.

In conclusion, colleges and universities are increasingly offering accommodations and support services to meet the needs of students with ADHD. Disability services, academic coaching, counseling services, study groups, assistive technology, peer mentoring, support groups, and flexibility with attendance and deadlines are all examples of accommodations and support services available to students with ADHD in higher education. It is essential for students with ADHD to take advantage of these resources to succeed in college. By seeking out support and accommodations, students with ADHD can thrive in college and achieve their academic goals.

Tips for academic success and managing stress

For students with ADHD, academic success can often be a challenge. ADHD can make it difficult to stay organized, manage time effectively, and stay focused on tasks. However, with the right strategies and support, students with ADHD can achieve academic success and manage stress. Below we will we will explore some tips for academic success and managing stress for students with ADHD.

1. Use a Planner or Calendar: One of the most effective strategies for managing time and staying organized is to use a planner or calendar. Students with ADHD can benefit from having a visual representation of their schedule and assignments, which can help them stay on track and prioritize their time effectively.

2. Break Tasks into Smaller Pieces: Students with ADHD may become overwhelmed by large assignments or projects. Breaking these tasks into smaller, more manageable pieces can make them feel less daunting and more achievable.

3. Develop Effective Study Habits: Effective study habits can help students with ADHD stay focused and engaged during study sessions. Some effective study habits include using active learning techniques, such as taking notes or creating study guides, and studying in a distraction-free environment.

4. Take Breaks: Students with ADHD may become restless or unfocused if they try to work for long periods without breaks. Taking short breaks every 30-45 minutes can help students stay focused and avoid burnout.

5. Use Accommodations: Accommodations, such as extended time on tests or note-taking services, can help students with ADHD succeed academically. It is important for students with ADHD to work with their school's disability services office to identify and implement appropriate accommodations.

6. Develop Coping Strategies: Coping strategies can help students with ADHD manage stress and maintain a healthy work-life balance. Some effective coping strategies include exercise, mindfulness meditation, and time management strategies.

7. Seek Support: Students with ADHD may benefit from seeking support from peers, family members, or mental health professionals. Support can help students feel less isolated and overwhelmed and can provide valuable guidance and encouragement.

8. Practice Self-Care: Practicing self-care is essential for managing stress and maintaining overall health and well-being. Some effective self-care strategies include getting enough sleep, eating a healthy diet, and engaging in activities that bring joy and relaxation.

In conclusion, academic success and stress management can be challenging for students with ADHD, but with the right strategies and support, it is achievable. Using a planner or calendar, breaking tasks into smaller pieces, developing effective study habits, taking breaks, using accommodations, developing coping strategies, seeking support, and practicing self-care are all effective strategies for managing ADHD and achieving academic success. By incorporating these strategies into their daily routine, students with ADHD can thrive academically and manage stress more effectively.

Chapter Ten

ADHD and the Workplace

Attention Deficit Hyperactivity Disorder (ADHD) can affect individuals in various areas of life, including the workplace. ADHD can make it challenging to stay organized, focus on tasks, and manage time effectively, which can impact job performance and success. However, with the right strategies and support, individuals with ADHD can succeed in the workplace. Below we will we will explore some tips for navigating the workplace with ADHD.

1. Seek Accommodations: Individuals with ADHD may benefit from requesting accommodations in the workplace. Accommodations can include things like flexible scheduling, frequent breaks, and noise-cancelling headphones. Accommodations can help individuals with ADHD manage their symptoms and improve job performance.

2. Develop Effective Time Management Strategies: Time management can be a challenge for individuals with ADHD. Developing effective time management strategies, such as breaking tasks into smaller pieces, prioritizing tasks, and using a planner or calendar, can help individuals with ADHD stay on track and meet deadlines.

3. Minimize Distractions: Individuals with ADHD may be more susceptible to distractions in the workplace. Minimizing distractions, such as turning off notifications on phones and computers, can help individuals with ADHD stay focused on tasks.

4. Communicate with Coworkers and Supervisors: Communication is key in the workplace, especially for individuals with ADHD. Communicating with coworkers and supervisors about one's ADHD and any necessary accommodations can help create a supportive work environment.

5. Use Technology: Technology can be a helpful tool for individuals with ADHD in the workplace. There are numerous apps and tools available that can help with time management, organization, and productivity.

6. Take Breaks: Taking breaks throughout the workday can be beneficial for individuals with ADHD. Short breaks can help individuals stay focused and reduce stress levels.

7. Develop Coping Strategies: Coping strategies can help individuals with ADHD manage stress and maintain a healthy work-life balance. Some effective coping strategies include exercise, mindfulness meditation, and time management strategies.

8. Seek Support: Individuals with ADHD may benefit from seeking support from a mental health professional or ADHD coach. Support can help individuals with ADHD manage their symptoms and develop effective strategies for succeeding in the workplace.

In conclusion, ADHD can pose challenges in the workplace, but with the right strategies and support, individuals with ADHD can succeed. Seeking accommodations, developing effective time management strategies, minimizing distractions, communicating with coworkers and supervisors, using technology, taking breaks, developing coping strategies, and seeking support are all effective strategies for navigating the workplace with ADHD. By incorporating these strategies into their work routine, individuals with ADHD can thrive in their careers and achieve success in the workplace.

Disclosing ADHD in the workplace

Attention Deficit Hyperactivity Disorder (ADHD) is a neurodevelopmental disorder that affects an individual's ability to focus, organize, and manage time effectively. While ADHD can present challenges in various areas of life, it can be particularly challenging in the workplace. Individuals with ADHD may struggle with tasks such as staying organized, prioritizing tasks, and meeting deadlines, which can impact job performance and success. Disclosing ADHD in the workplace is a personal decision that requires careful consideration. Below we will we will explore the pros and cons of disclosing ADHD in the workplace and provide some tips for individuals with ADHD who are considering disclosing their diagnosis.

Pros of Disclosing ADHD in the Workplace:

1. Accommodations: Disclosing ADHD in the workplace can lead to accommodations that can help individuals with ADHD manage their symptoms and improve job performance. Accommodations can include things like flexible scheduling, frequent breaks, and noise-cancelling headphones.

2. Support: Disclosing ADHD can also lead to support from coworkers and supervisors. Coworkers and supervisors who understand an individual's ADHD may be more supportive and accommodating.

3. Improved Communication: Disclosing ADHD can lead to improved communication in the workplace. Coworkers and supervisors who understand an individual's ADHD may be more patient and understanding when communicating with them.

4. Increased Understanding: Disclosing ADHD can also increase understanding of the disorder in the workplace. By disclosing their ADHD, individuals can help reduce stigma and increase awareness of the disorder.

Cons of Disclosing ADHD in the Workplace:

5. Discrimination: Disclosing ADHD in the workplace can lead to discrimination, such as being passed over for promotions or being treated unfairly by coworkers or supervisors.

6. Stigma: Disclosing ADHD can also lead to stigma and negative attitudes from coworkers or supervisors who do not understand the disorder.

7. Privacy Concerns: Disclosing ADHD can also lead to privacy concerns, as an individual's ADHD diagnosis becomes part of their employment record.

Tips for Disclosing ADHD in the Workplace:

8. Consider the Risks and Benefits: When deciding whether to disclose their ADHD in the workplace, individuals should carefully consider the risks and benefits. If the benefits outweigh the risks, disclosing ADHD may be a good decision.

9. Choose the Right Time and Place: It is important to choose the right time and place to disclose ADHD in the workplace. A private meeting with a supervisor or HR representative may be the best option.

10. Be Prepared: When disclosing ADHD, individuals should be prepared to explain the disorder and how it affects their work. They should also be prepared to provide information about any necessary accommodations.

11. Focus on the Positive: When disclosing ADHD, it is important to focus on the positive aspects of the disorder, such as creativity and problem-solving skills.

12. Seek Support: Individuals with ADHD who are considering disclosing their diagnosis may benefit from seeking support from a mental health professional or ADHD coach.

In conclusion, disclosing ADHD in the workplace is a personal decision that requires careful consideration. While there are risks and benefits to disclosing ADHD, individuals can take steps to minimize the risks and increase the benefits. Considering the risks and benefits, choosing the right time and place, being prepared, focusing on the positive, and seeking support are all effective strategies for individuals with ADHD who are considering disclosing their diagnosis in the workplace. By carefully considering their options and taking steps to protect their privacy and job security, individuals with ADHD can thrive in the workplace and achieve success in their careers.

Workplace accommodations and strategies for success

Attention-deficit/hyperactivity disorder (ADHD) is a neurodevelopmental disorder that affects both children and adults. While ADHD is commonly associated with academic settings, it can also have a significant impact on the workplace. Individuals with ADHD may experience difficulties with attention, organization, time management, and impulse control, which can impact their work performance and interpersonal relationships with colleagues. Fortunately, with the right accommodations and strategies, individuals with ADHD can successfully navigate the workplace.

The Americans with Disabilities Act (ADA) prohibits discrimination against individuals with disabilities in the workplace, including those with ADHD. This means that individuals with ADHD have a legal right to request reasonable accommodations from their employer. Accommodations can vary depending on the specific needs of the individual, but may include flexible work hours, the ability to work from home, noise-cancelling headphones, and written rather than verbal instructions.

In addition to accommodations, there are several strategies that individuals with ADHD can use to improve their work performance. One key strategy is to prioritize tasks and break them down into smaller, manageable steps. This can help individuals with ADHD avoid feeling overwhelmed and ensure that important tasks are completed on time. Additionally, individuals with ADHD may benefit from using timers or alarms to help them stay on track and avoid getting lost in hyperfocus.

Another effective strategy is to use organizational tools such as to-do lists, calendars, and project management software. These tools can help individuals with ADHD keep track of deadlines, appointments, and important tasks. It can also be helpful to create a designated workspace that is free from distractions and has all necessary supplies readily available.

Communication with colleagues and supervisors is also important for individuals with ADHD. It can be helpful to explain ADHD symptoms and how they may impact work performance to colleagues and supervisors. This can help colleagues better understand why an individual may struggle with certain tasks and may encourage a more supportive and understanding work environment. Additionally, individuals with ADHD may benefit from regular check-ins with their supervisor to ensure that they are staying on track and to address any challenges or concerns that arise.

In addition to accommodations and strategies, it is important for individuals with ADHD to prioritize self-care in the workplace. This includes getting enough sleep, staying physically active, and maintaining a healthy diet. It is also important to take breaks throughout the workday to reduce stress and prevent burnout.

Disclosing ADHD in the workplace can be a difficult decision for many individuals. While the ADA protects individuals with disabilities from discrimination, there may still be stigma associated with ADHD in some workplace settings. Ultimately, the decision to disclose ADHD should be based on an individual's specific circumstances and comfort level. It may be helpful to consult with a healthcare provider or a human resources representative before making a decision.

In conclusion, ADHD can have a significant impact on the workplace, but with the right accommodations and strategies, individuals with ADHD can succeed. It is important for individuals with ADHD to understand their legal rights and to advocate for themselves in the workplace. By prioritizing self-care, effective communication, and organizational strategies, individuals with ADHD can thrive in the workplace and achieve their professional goals.

Navigating career challenges and transitions

Navigating Career Challenges and Transitions with ADHD

Attention Deficit Hyperactivity Disorder (ADHD) can present unique challenges in the workplace, particularly when it comes to career advancement and transitions. Individuals with ADHD may struggle with time management, organization, and maintaining focus on tasks. These difficulties can affect job performance, hinder professional growth, and create barriers to new opportunities.

However, with the right strategies and support, individuals with ADHD can successfully navigate career challenges and transitions. Below we will we will explore the impact of ADHD on career success, provide tips for overcoming career obstacles, and discuss strategies for transitioning to new career opportunities.

The Impact of ADHD on Career Success

ADHD can have a significant impact on career success, particularly in fields that require a high level of focus, organization, and time management skills. For individuals with ADHD, these skills can be particularly challenging, leading to decreased productivity, missed deadlines, and difficulties with communication.

In addition, individuals with ADHD may struggle with interpersonal skills, which can impact relationships with colleagues, managers, and clients. For example, individuals with ADHD may have difficulty with social cues, communication, and maintaining appropriate levels of engagement in group settings.

Despite these challenges, many individuals with ADHD are successful in their careers. In fact, some research suggests that individuals with ADHD may have unique strengths that can be beneficial in certain fields. For example, individuals with ADHD may excel in creative fields, such as writing, graphic design, or advertising, due to their ability to think outside the box and generate new ideas.

Tips for Overcoming Career Obstacles

Individuals with ADHD can take steps to overcome career obstacles and achieve success in their chosen field. Here are some tips for navigating the challenges of ADHD in the workplace:

1. Build a strong support network: Having a supportive manager, mentor, or colleague can be invaluable for individuals with ADHD. Seek out individuals who can provide guidance, feedback, and support as needed.

2. Develop strong organizational and time management skills: Individuals with ADHD can benefit from developing strong organizational and time management skills. This may involve using tools such as calendars, to-do lists, and reminders to stay on top of deadlines and responsibilities.

3. Find ways to stay focused and engaged: Individuals with ADHD may benefit from finding ways to stay engaged and focused on tasks, such as

breaking work into smaller, manageable tasks, using visual aids to stay on track, or setting goals and rewards for completing tasks.

4. Communicate openly with colleagues and managers: Communication is key in any workplace, but it is particularly important for individuals with ADHD. Be open about your strengths and weaknesses, and communicate your needs and preferences as appropriate.

Strategies for Transitioning to New Career Opportunities

Transitioning to a new career can be challenging for anyone, but individuals with ADHD may face additional obstacles. However, with the right strategies and support, individuals with ADHD can successfully navigate career transitions. Here are some tips for transitioning to a new career:

5. Assess your strengths and interests: When considering a new career, it is important to assess your strengths and interests. Consider what tasks and activities you enjoy, and what comes naturally to you.

6. Seek out opportunities for skill-building and training: If there are areas where you feel you could improve your skills, seek out opportunities for training and skill-building. This may involve taking classes, attending workshops, or seeking out mentors in your chosen field.

7. Network and build connections: Networking is an important part of any career transition. Reach out to colleagues, alumni from your college or university, and others in your chosen field to build connections and learn about new opportunities.

8. Be open to new experiences and opportunities: Career transitions often involve stepping outside of your comfort zone and taking on new challenges. Be open to new experiences and opportunities, and embrace the learning process

Chapter Eleven

ADHD and Relationships

Attention Deficit Hyperactivity Disorder (ADHD) is a neurodevelopmental disorder that affects people of all ages. It can impact many areas of life, including relationships with others. Individuals with ADHD may struggle with social skills, communication, and managing their emotions, which can cause challenges in personal and professional relationships. However, with understanding and support, people with ADHD can develop successful relationships and thrive.

ADHD and Relationships

Attention and impulse control are two key components of ADHD. People with ADHD may struggle to pay attention to conversations, follow through with plans or promises, or regulate their emotions. These symptoms can make it difficult to build and maintain strong relationships, as communication and reliability are crucial components of healthy relationships.

People with ADHD may also struggle with social cues and picking up on non-verbal communication. This can make it challenging to understand the emotions of others and to respond appropriately. They may also have difficulty regulating their own emotions, leading to impulsivity and outbursts that can cause strain on relationships.

In addition, the symptoms of ADHD can make it challenging to balance the demands of work and home life, leading to additional stress and strain on relationships. These challenges can cause misunderstandings, conflict, and even relationship breakdowns if not properly addressed.

Supporting Relationships with ADHD

Despite the challenges, people with ADHD can develop healthy and successful relationships with support and guidance. The following are some strategies that can be helpful:

1. Education and understanding: Education is key to understanding the challenges and strengths of ADHD. Both individuals with ADHD and their partners can benefit from learning about the disorder, its symptoms, and how it affects relationships.

2. Open communication: Communication is critical to the success of any relationship, but especially important when one or both partners have ADHD. Regular, open communication can help to reduce misunderstandings and increase understanding and support.

3. Structure and routine: Creating structure and routine in daily life can help to reduce the impact of ADHD symptoms on relationships. This can include setting regular schedules for activities, such as meal times and bedtimes, as well as creating systems for organizing and managing tasks and responsibilities.

4. Counseling: Couples counseling or individual therapy can be a helpful tool for addressing relationship challenges related to ADHD. A therapist can provide guidance and support to help couples build effective communication skills, work through conflict, and develop strategies for managing ADHD symptoms.

5. Medication and other treatments: Medication and other treatments can be effective in reducing the symptoms of ADHD and improving overall

functioning, which can help to reduce the impact of ADHD on relationships.

6. Support groups: Support groups can provide a sense of community and understanding for individuals and families affected by ADHD. They can also offer practical advice and tips for managing the challenges of the disorder.

Conclusion

ADHD can pose challenges to relationships, but with understanding, support, and effective strategies, people with ADHD can build successful and fulfilling relationships with their partners, friends, and family. Communication, education, structure, counseling, medication, and support groups can all be helpful tools in managing the symptoms of ADHD and building strong relationships.

The impact of ADHD on romantic relationships and friendships

Attention Deficit Hyperactivity Disorder (ADHD) can have a significant impact on an individual's social life, including their romantic relationships and friendships. ADHD is a neurodevelopmental disorder characterized by symptoms of inattention, hyperactivity, and impulsivity. While these symptoms can be challenging in many areas of life, they can create unique difficulties in interpersonal relationships.

In romantic relationships, ADHD symptoms can interfere with communication and create misunderstandings between partners. For example, an individual with ADHD may struggle to listen actively or may frequently interrupt their partner. They may also struggle with maintaining focus during conversations or completing tasks related to the relationship, such as planning dates or remembering important dates. These challenges can lead to frustration and conflict in the relationship.

Additionally, individuals with ADHD may struggle with managing emotions, which can lead to mood swings, outbursts, and difficulty regulating reactions to stress or conflict. This can make it challenging for partners to navigate difficult conversations or disagreements, and can create tension in the relationship.

ADHD can also have an impact on friendships, as individuals with ADHD may struggle with social skills such as listening, sharing, and taking turns in conversation. They may struggle to read social cues and may not pick up on nonverbal communication, leading to misunderstandings or missed social cues. This can make it difficult to form and maintain friendships, especially with those who do not understand or accommodate for their symptoms.

However, with understanding and support, individuals with ADHD can have successful relationships and friendships. Open communication and honesty are key components in romantic relationships, and individuals with ADHD can work to develop strategies for managing their symptoms, such as using tools like calendars or reminders to keep track of important dates or commitments. Couples therapy can also be a helpful tool for improving communication and addressing conflicts in the relationship.

In friendships, individuals with ADHD can benefit from finding social outlets that allow them to connect with others who understand or accommodate for their symptoms. They can also work to develop social skills through therapies such as cognitive-behavioral therapy or social skills training.

It's important to note that while ADHD can create unique challenges in interpersonal relationships, it's not a guarantee that individuals with

ADHD will struggle in these areas. Every individual is different, and the severity of symptoms and their impact on relationships can vary widely.

It's also important to remember that relationships and friendships are a two-way street, and both parties must be willing to put in effort and work to maintain a healthy dynamic. Partners and friends of individuals with ADHD can also work to educate themselves about the disorder and develop strategies for supporting their loved one.

In summary, ADHD can have a significant impact on romantic relationships and friendships due to challenges with communication, emotional regulation, and social skills. However, with understanding and support, individuals with ADHD can have successful relationships and friendships. Open communication, honesty, and developing strategies for managing symptoms are key components in navigating interpersonal relationships with ADHD. Additionally, partners and friends can work to educate themselves about the disorder and develop strategies for supporting their loved one.

Communication strategies for healthy relationships

Communication is the foundation of any healthy relationship, and this is particularly true when one or both partners have ADHD. ADHD can present unique challenges in communication, such as difficulties with staying focused, listening actively, and regulating emotions. However, with some intentional effort and practice, individuals with ADHD can develop effective communication strategies that enhance their relationships.

One strategy for effective communication is to set clear expectations and boundaries. This can involve establishing guidelines for communication, such as designating specific times for checking in with each other, or outlining how conflicts will be resolved. Clear expectations and boundaries can help both partners understand what is expected of them, reduce misunderstandings, and provide a sense of security within the relationship.

Another important strategy is to actively listen to each other. For individuals with ADHD, this can be particularly challenging, as their minds may be racing with other thoughts or distractions. However, active listening involves paying full attention to the other person, asking clarifying questions, and summarizing what was said to ensure understanding. By practicing active listening, individuals with ADHD can improve their communication skills and build stronger relationships.

It is also important to be aware of nonverbal communication, such as facial expressions and body language. Individuals with ADHD may struggle with interpreting nonverbal cues, so it can be helpful to discuss these cues with their partners and to practice recognizing them. Additionally, being mindful of one's own nonverbal communication can help to convey the intended message and avoid unintentional misunderstandings.

In addition to these strategies, individuals with ADHD may benefit from seeking support from a therapist or coach who specializes in ADHD and relationships. These professionals can provide guidance on communication skills and offer strategies for managing symptoms of ADHD that may impact communication.

Friendships can also be impacted by ADHD, particularly when individuals with ADHD struggle with social skills and maintaining connections with others. However, there are strategies that can help individuals with ADHD build and maintain friendships.

One strategy is to focus on shared interests or hobbies. This can provide a common ground for individuals with ADHD to connect with others and develop friendships. Additionally, individuals with ADHD can work on developing social skills, such as active listening and empathy, through practice and guidance from a therapist or coach.

Another important strategy is to be open and honest about one's struggles with ADHD. This can help to reduce stigma and create a safe space for individuals with ADHD to connect with others who may also be struggling with similar challenges. Additionally, being upfront about ADHD can help to manage expectations in friendships, such as explaining that it may be difficult to respond to messages in a timely manner or to attend social events.

In conclusion, effective communication is key to building and maintaining healthy relationships, and this is particularly true when one or both partners have ADHD. By practicing strategies such as setting clear expectations, active listening, and being aware of nonverbal communication, individuals with ADHD can improve their communication skills and enhance their relationships. Additionally, seeking support from a therapist or coach who specializes in ADHD and relationships can be helpful in developing effective communication strategies. For friendships, focusing on shared interests, developing social skills, and being open and honest about one's struggles with ADHD can help individuals with ADHD build and maintain meaningful connections with others.

Building and maintaining a strong support network

Attention-deficit/hyperactivity disorder (ADHD) can significantly impact a person's daily life, including their relationships with others. Having a strong support network is essential for individuals with ADHD to manage their symptoms and navigate the challenges that may arise. Below we will we will discuss strategies for building and maintaining a strong support network for those with ADHD.

One of the most important strategies for building a support network is identifying and connecting with others who understand what it's like to live with ADHD. This may include seeking out support groups, both in-person and online. Support groups can provide a safe and non-judgmental space to share experiences and coping strategies, as well as receive emotional support and encouragement from others who are going through similar challenges.

Another important component of building a support network is reaching out to family and friends. Educating loved ones about ADHD and how it affects you can help them better understand your experiences and provide the support you need. It's important to communicate openly and honestly with loved ones about your struggles, but also celebrate your strengths and accomplishments.

In addition to support groups and loved ones, seeking out professional help can also be beneficial. This may include therapy, coaching, or medication management with a healthcare provider. A mental health professional can help individuals with ADHD develop coping strategies, manage symptoms, and address any underlying emotional or mental health concerns.

Technology can also be a useful tool for building a support network. Social media and online forums can connect individuals with ADHD with others who share similar experiences and interests. There are also numerous apps and tools designed specifically for managing ADHD symptoms, such as organization and productivity apps, meditation and mindfulness apps, and medication tracking tools.

It's important to remember that building a support network is an ongoing process and requires effort and commitment. It's important to stay connected with loved ones, attend support group meetings regularly, and continue therapy or coaching as needed. It's also important to be open to trying new strategies and seeking out additional support when necessary.

Maintaining a strong support network also requires effective communication and boundaries. It's important to communicate your needs and boundaries with loved ones and support group members. This may include setting boundaries around social events, work commitments, or other activities that may be overwhelming or triggering for individuals with ADHD. It's also important to communicate with loved ones about any changes in treatment or medication, as this can impact mood and behavior.

In addition to setting boundaries, it's important to engage in self-care practices to manage stress and prevent burnout. This may include exercise, meditation, getting enough sleep, and engaging in hobbies or activities that bring joy and relaxation.

In conclusion, building and maintaining a strong support network is essential for individuals with ADHD to manage their symptoms and thrive in their daily lives. This may include joining support groups, seeking professional help, connecting with loved ones, and utilizing technology. Effective communication, setting boundaries, and engaging in self-care practices are also important strategies for maintaining a strong support network. With the right support and resources, individuals with ADHD can live fulfilling and successful lives.

Chapter Twelve

Parenting a Child with ADHD

Parenting a child with ADHD can be a challenging experience, but with the right strategies and support, it is possible to create a nurturing and stable environment for your child. ADHD, or attention deficit hyperactivity disorder, is a neurodevelopmental disorder that affects a child's ability to focus, organize, and manage their behavior. Below we will we will discuss some tips and strategies for parenting a child with ADHD.

Educate Yourself

One of the most important things you can do as a parent of a child with ADHD is to educate yourself about the disorder. Learn about the symptoms, causes, and treatments of ADHD. Understanding your child's condition will help you better support them and advocate for their needs. You can seek information from reputable sources such as the National Institute of Mental Health or reputable medical journals.

Work with a Healthcare Professional

It is important to work with a healthcare professional who specializes in ADHD to help manage your child's condition. This may include a pediatrician, psychiatrist, or psychologist. A healthcare professional can help determine the appropriate medication and dosage for your child and recommend behavioral therapy or other interventions. Regular visits to the healthcare provider can help monitor your child's progress and ensure they are receiving the appropriate care.

Create a Structured Environment

Children with ADHD often benefit from structure and routine. Create a structured environment at home by setting up a daily routine and sticking to it. Consistent routines help children with ADHD manage their behavior and reduce stress. This may include consistent times for meals, homework, and bedtime. It is also helpful to create a calm and quiet space for your child to work on homework or play.

Set Clear Expectations and Consequences

Children with ADHD may struggle with impulse control and behavior management. Setting clear expectations and consequences can help your child understand what is expected of them and how their behavior will be managed. Use clear and concise language when setting expectations and use positive reinforcement when your child meets expectations. For example, praise your child for completing homework on time or following directions. Use age-appropriate consequences for misbehavior, such as a time-out or loss of privileges.

Encourage Positive Behavior

Children with ADHD may struggle with self-esteem and self-worth due to the challenges they face. Encourage positive behavior by acknowledging and praising your child's strengths and accomplishments. Celebrate successes, no matter how small, and provide opportunities for your child to succeed in areas they are interested in. Positive reinforcement can help boost your child's self-esteem and create a more positive outlook.

Communicate with Teachers and Other Caregivers

It is important to communicate with your child's teachers and other caregivers to ensure they understand your child's needs and can provide the appropriate support. This may include accommodations in the classroom, such as extra time for assignments or preferential seating. You can also provide resources and information to caregivers, such as books or websites, to help them better understand ADHD.

Take Care of Yourself

Parenting a child with ADHD can be stressful and challenging. It is important to take care of yourself to ensure you have the energy and resources to care for your child. This may include taking breaks when needed, seeking support from family and friends, and practicing self-care activities such as exercise or meditation.

In conclusion, parenting a child with ADHD requires patience, understanding, and support. Educating yourself, working with healthcare professionals, creating a structured environment, setting clear expectations, encouraging positive behavior, communicating with caregivers, and taking care of yourself are all important strategies for parenting a child with ADHD. With the right strategies and support, you can help your child thrive and succeed.

Understanding the unique challenges of raising a child with ADHD

Attention Deficit Hyperactivity Disorder (ADHD) is a neurodevelopmental disorder that affects millions of children worldwide. Parenting a child with ADHD presents a unique set of challenges for caregivers, as the condition can cause behavioral and academic difficulties that may require specialized attention. Understanding the disorder and its effects on the child is crucial for effective management and positive outcomes. Below we will we will discuss the unique challenges of raising a child with ADHD and explore strategies for successful parenting.

One of the primary challenges faced by parents of children with ADHD is managing the symptoms of the disorder. The core symptoms of ADHD include inattention, hyperactivity, and impulsivity, and can manifest in various ways. Children with ADHD may have difficulty focusing on tasks or following instructions, experience restlessness or excessive movement, and may act impulsively without considering the consequences of their actions. These symptoms can cause academic difficulties, social problems, and increased risk for injury.

Another challenge is the stigma surrounding ADHD. Children with ADHD may be stigmatized by peers or adults who misunderstand the disorder and its effects on behavior. Parents may also feel judged or blamed for their child's behavior, which can lead to feelings of shame or inadequacy. Addressing these stigmas through education and advocacy can help create a more supportive environment for families of children with ADHD.

Effective management of ADHD requires a comprehensive approach that includes various interventions and strategies. One important strategy is behavioral therapy, which teaches children coping skills and helps them develop positive habits and routines. Parent training can also be an effective tool for improving the parent-child relationship and addressing problematic behaviors. In addition, medication may be prescribed to help manage symptoms, but this should always be done in consultation with a qualified healthcare professional.

Parents of children with ADHD should also focus on creating a supportive environment at home. This includes establishing routines and clear expectations, providing positive reinforcement, and offering emotional support. Parents should also communicate regularly with teachers and other caregivers to ensure consistency in managing the child's symptoms. This collaboration can also help identify areas where the child may need extra support, such as tutoring or accommodations in the classroom.

It is also important for parents to prioritize their own self-care. Raising a child with ADHD can be emotionally taxing, and parents may need support to manage stress and maintain their own well-being. This may include seeking counseling, joining a support group, or engaging in stress-reducing activities such as exercise or mindfulness practices.

In conclusion, parenting a child with ADHD presents unique challenges that require specialized attention and strategies. Effective management of the disorder involves a comprehensive approach that includes medication, behavioral therapy, parent training, and supportive home environments. Addressing stigmas and prioritizing self-care are also important for successful parenting. By understanding the disorder and its effects on behavior, parents can help their child reach their full potential and thrive.

Strategies for managing behavior and promoting success

ADHD, or Attention Deficit Hyperactivity Disorder, can present unique challenges for parents when it comes to managing their child's behavior and promoting success in school and social settings. While every child with ADHD is unique, there are several strategies that can be effective in managing behavior and setting them up for success.

One key strategy is to establish clear and consistent routines. Children with ADHD often benefit from having a structured routine, as it can help them stay on task and reduce their level of anxiety. This routine can include specific times for meals, homework, and leisure activities, and can be written down or displayed visually to help them stay organized.

Another important strategy is to set clear expectations and consequences for behavior. This can involve establishing clear rules for behavior and outlining the consequences for breaking them, such as losing privileges or having to do extra chores. Consistency is key here, as children with ADHD may struggle with impulse control and need consistent reminders of what is expected of them.

Parents can also work with their child's school to develop a plan for accommodations and support. This may include accommodations such as extra time on tests or preferential seating in the classroom. Additionally, parents can work with their child's teacher to establish a system of rewards for positive behavior, such as a sticker chart or small prizes for meeting goals.

It's also important to help children with ADHD develop self-regulation skills. This can include strategies such as deep breathing, taking breaks when feeling overwhelmed, and learning to identify and manage their emotions. Parents can work with their child to develop a list of coping strategies that they can use when feeling anxious or overwhelmed.

Finally, it's important for parents to take care of themselves as well. Raising a child with ADHD can be stressful, and it's important for parents to practice self-care and seek support when needed. This can include taking breaks when needed, reaching out to other parents of children with ADHD for support, or seeking professional help when necessary.

In conclusion, parenting a child with ADHD can present unique challenges, but there are several strategies that can be effective in managing behavior and promoting success. These strategies include establishing clear and consistent routines, setting clear expectations and consequences for behavior, working with the school to develop accommodations and support, helping children develop self-regulation skills, and practicing self-care as a parent. By implementing these strategies, parents can help their child with ADHD thrive and succeed in all areas of life.

Self-care for parents of children with ADHD

Self-care for parents of children with ADHD

Raising a child with Attention Deficit Hyperactivity Disorder (ADHD) can be challenging and overwhelming for parents. Children with ADHD may have difficulty with impulse control, hyperactivity, and inattention, which can make parenting them more demanding. As a result, it is important for parents to practice self-care to ensure that they are equipped to handle the challenges that come with parenting a child with ADHD. Below we will we will discuss the importance of self-care for parents of children with ADHD and strategies that can be used to manage the stress and challenges of raising a child with ADHD.

The Importance of Self-Care for Parents of Children with ADHD

Parents of children with ADHD often find themselves with additional responsibilities, such as scheduling doctor appointments, attending therapy sessions, and providing additional support to their children. The added demands of raising a child with ADHD can be exhausting and can take a toll on a parent's physical and emotional well-being. Therefore, it is essential for parents to prioritize their own self-care to ensure they are equipped to manage the challenges that come with parenting a child with ADHD.

Self-care can help parents to manage stress, avoid burnout, and reduce feelings of frustration and exhaustion. By taking care of their own needs, parents can approach their child's needs with more patience and compassion, which can strengthen the parent-child relationship. Self-care can also promote positive mental health, which can help parents to be more resilient and better equipped to handle the ups and downs of parenting a child with ADHD.

Strategies for Self-Care for Parents of Children with ADHD

1. Prioritize Sleep: Parents of children with ADHD often have disrupted sleep patterns due to the demands of parenting. It is important for parents to prioritize sleep and aim for at least 7-8 hours of sleep per night. Creating a bedtime routine and sticking to a regular sleep schedule can help improve the quality of sleep and promote relaxation.

2. Engage in Physical Activity: Regular exercise can help to reduce stress and promote positive mental health. Parents can incorporate physical activity into their daily routine by taking a walk or bike ride with their child or attending a fitness class.

3. Seek Support: Parenting a child with ADHD can be isolating, and it is important for parents to seek support from others who can relate to their experience. Joining a support group, attending therapy, or talking to other parents who have experience with ADHD can provide validation and support.

4. Practice Mindfulness: Mindfulness techniques such as deep breathing, meditation, and yoga can help to reduce stress and promote relaxation. Parents can practice mindfulness techniques during moments of stress or anxiety throughout the day.

5. Make Time for Hobbies and Activities: Engaging in hobbies and activities can provide a sense of fulfillment and help to reduce stress. Parents can set aside time each week to engage in activities they enjoy, such as reading a book, painting, or cooking.

6. Take Breaks: It is important for parents to take breaks and engage in activities that are solely for their own enjoyment. Taking a few minutes to read a book or listen to music can provide a sense of relaxation and reduce stress.

7. Establish Boundaries: Parents of children with ADHD often feel pressure to be constantly available and accommodating to their child's needs. However, it is important for parents to establish boundaries and communicate their own needs. Saying no to additional responsibilities and delegating tasks can help to reduce stress and promote self-care.

Conclusion

Parenting a child with ADHD can be challenging and overwhelming, but prioritizing self-care can help parents to manage stress and promote positive mental health. By taking care of their own needs, parents can approach their child's needs with more patience and compassion, which can strengthen the parent-child relationship.

Chapter Thirteen

ADHD in Women and Girls

ADHD is a neurodevelopmental disorder that affects both males and females, but historically, the disorder has been primarily studied in males. It is only in recent years that researchers have begun to explore the unique manifestation of ADHD in women and girls. Below we will discuss ADHD in women and girls, including the prevalence, symptoms, and challenges faced by those with the disorder.

Prevalence:

According to the Centers for Disease Control and Prevention (CDC), approximately 6.1 million children in the United States have been diagnosed with ADHD. However, ADHD is not just a childhood disorder. The American Psychological Association estimates that 4% of adults in the United States have ADHD. The prevalence of ADHD in women and girls has historically been underestimated, with studies suggesting that females with ADHD are often underdiagnosed and undertreated. While the exact prevalence of ADHD in women and girls is unknown, research suggests that it may be as high as 5% of the female population.

Symptoms:

ADHD symptoms in females can differ from those in males. While hyperactivity is often more prominent in males with ADHD, females may present with inattentive symptoms. For example, girls with ADHD may be daydreamy, forgetful, and disorganized. They may have trouble completing tasks, lose things frequently, and struggle with time management. These symptoms may be misattributed to laziness or a lack of motivation, rather than an underlying neurological condition.

In addition to inattention, women and girls with ADHD may also experience emotional dysregulation. This can manifest as mood swings, anxiety, depression, and low self-esteem. Girls with ADHD may be more prone to social rejection and may struggle to form and maintain friendships.

Challenges:

The challenges faced by women and girls with ADHD are unique and can have a significant impact on their daily lives. Many women with ADHD report feeling overwhelmed and burnt out by the demands of work, school, and household responsibilities. Women with ADHD may struggle to prioritize tasks and may feel guilty or ashamed when they are unable to complete tasks on time.

Women and girls with ADHD may also face stigma and discrimination. ADHD is often viewed as a disorder that primarily affects boys and men, leading to the underdiagnosis and undertreatment of females with the disorder. Women and girls with ADHD may be judged harshly for their symptoms, with their behavior being attributed to personality flaws rather than a neurodevelopmental disorder.

Treatment:

The treatment of ADHD in women and girls is similar to that of males with the disorder. This typically involves a combination of medication and behavioral therapy. However, there are some unique considerations when treating females with ADHD. For example, some women may be hesitant to take medication due to concerns about pregnancy and breastfeeding.

Additionally, women with ADHD may require additional support to manage the demands of work and family life.

Conclusion:

ADHD is a complex disorder that affects both males and females, although the presentation of symptoms can differ between the two genders. Women and girls with ADHD often face unique challenges, including underdiagnosis, undertreatment, and stigma. The effective management of ADHD in females requires a comprehensive approach that considers the unique needs and challenges faced by these individuals. With proper treatment and support, women and girls with ADHD can thrive and achieve their goals.

Unique presentation and challenges of ADHD in females

Attention-deficit/hyperactivity disorder (ADHD) is commonly thought of as a disorder that primarily affects boys and men. However, recent research has revealed that ADHD is just as prevalent in girls and women. The disorder presents differently in females, making it more difficult to diagnose and treat. Below we will we will discuss the unique presentation and challenges of ADHD in females.

1. According to the Centers for Disease Control and Prevention (CDC), approximately 11% of American children between the ages of 4 and 17 have been diagnosed with ADHD. Boys are diagnosed with ADHD at a much higher rate than girls, with a ratio of 2:1. However, recent studies suggest that the ratio may be closer to 1.6:1. This indicates that girls may be underdiagnosed, as they often present with different symptoms than boys.

The most common symptoms of ADHD include inattention, hyperactivity, and impulsivity. Girls with ADHD tend to exhibit more inattentive symptoms, which are often overlooked. Girls may be seen as daydreamers, spacey, or disorganized, rather than hyperactive or disruptive. They may be quiet and shy, leading others to believe that they are simply unmotivated or not trying hard enough.

Girls with ADHD are more likely to have problems with organization and time management, which can impact their academic and social lives. They may have difficulty completing tasks, forget to turn in homework, or struggle to maintain friendships. Girls with ADHD are also at a higher risk for anxiety and depression.

Another challenge in diagnosing ADHD in girls is the societal pressure to conform to gender norms. Girls are expected to be quiet, polite, and well-behaved, which can make it difficult for them to receive a diagnosis. This pressure can also lead to girls feeling ashamed or embarrassed about their symptoms and hesitant to seek help.

Treatment for ADHD in girls is similar to treatment for boys. Medication and behavioral therapy are effective in managing symptoms. However, it is important to note that girls with ADHD may require different dosages of medication than boys, as they tend to be smaller in size. Behavioral therapy can be especially helpful in teaching girls with ADHD skills to manage their symptoms and build self-esteem.

In addition to medication and therapy, lifestyle changes can also help manage symptoms of ADHD in girls. Regular exercise, a healthy diet, and good sleep habits can all be beneficial. Girls with ADHD may also benefit from participating in activities that allow them to focus their energy and attention, such as sports, music, or art.

In conclusion, ADHD is not just a disorder that affects boys and men. Girls and women can also have ADHD, but they often present with different symptoms than boys. Girls with ADHD may struggle with organization and time management, leading to academic and social difficulties. They may also be at a higher risk for anxiety and depression. The societal pressure to conform to gender norms can make it difficult for girls to receive a diagnosis and seek help. Treatment for ADHD in girls is similar to treatment for boys, but may require different dosages of medication. Lifestyle changes, such as exercise and healthy eating habits, can also be beneficial. It is important to recognize and address the unique challenges of ADHD in females to ensure they receive appropriate treatment and support.

Diagnosis and treatment considerations for women and girls

Attention-deficit/hyperactivity disorder (ADHD) is a neurodevelopmental condition that affects individuals across their lifespan. It is often characterized by symptoms such as inattention, hyperactivity, and impulsivity. While ADHD is often thought of as a condition that primarily affects boys and men, recent research has shown that it is also prevalent in girls and women, albeit often undiagnosed and underdiagnosed. Below we will we will explore the unique presentation and challenges of ADHD in females, as well as diagnosis and treatment considerations.

Historically, ADHD has been considered a condition that primarily affects boys and men. This perception is due in part to the fact that ADHD was initially studied and defined based on the behavior of hyperactive boys. However, more recent research has shown that ADHD is equally prevalent in girls and women. In fact, the National Institute of Mental

Health estimates that approximately 4.4% of adult women in the United States have ADHD.

One of the reasons ADHD is often overlooked in females is that it can present differently than it does in males. While hyperactivity and impulsivity are often more evident in males, females with ADHD may present primarily with symptoms of inattention. This can lead to the misconception that females are less likely to have ADHD, when in fact they may simply be exhibiting different symptoms. Additionally, girls and women with ADHD may be better at masking their symptoms and adapting to their environment, which can make it more difficult for clinicians to recognize the condition.

Another challenge with diagnosing ADHD in females is that the diagnostic criteria were developed based on research conducted on males. This means that the criteria may not capture the unique ways in which ADHD presents in females. For example, the criteria may emphasize hyperactivity and impulsivity, while downplaying symptoms of inattention that are more common in females. This can lead to underdiagnosis and misdiagnosis of females with ADHD.

Once a diagnosis of ADHD is made in a female, treatment considerations may also be different than they would be for a male with ADHD. Research has shown that females with ADHD may be more likely to experience anxiety and depression than males with ADHD. This means that treatment plans may need to address not only the core symptoms of ADHD, but also any co-occurring anxiety and mood disorders.

Treatment options for ADHD in females are similar to those for males and may include medication, behavioral therapy, and lifestyle changes. However, medication options may need to be adjusted based on factors such as weight and menstrual cycle. Additionally, behavioral therapy may need to address gender-specific issues such as societal expectations and gender roles.

In terms of lifestyle changes, females with ADHD may benefit from additional support in areas such as time management, organization, and self-care. Research has shown that females with ADHD are more likely to experience difficulties with executive functioning, which can impact their ability to plan and complete tasks. Providing support in these areas can help females with ADHD better manage their symptoms and improve their quality of life.

In conclusion, ADHD is a condition that affects both males and females, although it may present differently in each gender. Females with ADHD may be more likely to exhibit symptoms of inattention, and may also be more likely to experience anxiety and depression than males with ADHD. Diagnosis and treatment considerations for females may need to take these differences into account, and treatment plans may need to be tailored to address gender-specific issues. With appropriate diagnosis and treatment, females with ADHD can manage their symptoms and lead fulfilling lives.

The impact of hormones and life transitions on ADHD symptoms

Attention-deficit/hyperactivity disorder (ADHD) is a neurodevelopmental condition that affects individuals across the lifespan. While ADHD is often associated with children, it is estimated that approximately 4.4% of adults in the United States have ADHD, with a slightly higher prevalence in women than men. ADHD symptoms can be exacerbated by various factors, including hormones and life transitions.

Hormones play a significant role in the development and regulation of ADHD symptoms. In women, the menstrual cycle can impact symptom severity. Some women report an increase in hyperactivity, impulsivity, and irritability during the premenstrual phase, while others experience a decrease in symptoms. The fluctuations in hormones during pregnancy and postpartum can also affect ADHD symptoms. Research suggests that symptoms may improve during pregnancy, potentially due to an increase in estrogen levels. However, some women report an increase in symptoms postpartum, which may be due to a decrease in estrogen levels. Hormonal contraceptives may also impact ADHD symptoms, with some studies suggesting that oral contraceptives may exacerbate symptoms, while others suggest that hormonal IUDs may improve symptoms.

Life transitions, such as starting college, entering the workforce, and becoming a parent, can also impact ADHD symptoms. College students with ADHD may struggle with increased demands for time management, organization, and study skills. The workplace may pose similar challenges, such as managing deadlines, completing tasks, and maintaining focus. Parents with ADHD may find that the demands of raising children exacerbate their symptoms, particularly during periods of stress or sleep deprivation.

The impact of hormones and life transitions on ADHD symptoms underscores the importance of tailored treatment for women with ADHD. Treatment may involve a combination of medication, therapy, and lifestyle modifications. Medication is often an effective treatment for ADHD symptoms, but the type and dosage of medication may need to be adjusted to account for hormonal changes. Therapy can also be helpful in developing coping strategies and improving executive functioning skills. Cognitive-behavioral therapy (CBT) is a type of therapy that focuses on identifying and changing negative patterns of thought and behavior, and it has been found to be particularly effective for ADHD.

In addition to medication and therapy, lifestyle modifications can also be helpful in managing ADHD symptoms during times of hormonal fluctuations or life transitions. Regular exercise has been found to improve symptoms of ADHD, and it can also help to reduce stress and improve sleep. A healthy diet that is rich in omega-3 fatty acids, whole grains, and lean protein can also support brain health and improve ADHD symptoms. Adequate sleep is also crucial for managing symptoms, and individuals with ADHD may need to prioritize sleep hygiene practices such as establishing a regular bedtime routine and minimizing screen time before bed.

In conclusion, the impact of hormones and life transitions on ADHD symptoms highlights the importance of personalized treatment for women with ADHD. Hormonal fluctuations and life transitions can exacerbate ADHD symptoms, but medication, therapy, and lifestyle modifications can be effective in managing symptoms during these times. Further research is needed to better understand the relationship between hormones and ADHD, and to develop more targeted treatments for women with ADHD.

Chapter Fourteen

ADHD and Aging

ADHD, or Attention Deficit Hyperactivity Disorder, is a neurodevelopmental disorder that is commonly associated with children and adolescents. However, ADHD can also affect adults, including older adults. In fact, recent studies suggest that ADHD symptoms may persist into adulthood in up to 70% of cases. This means that ADHD is not a condition that is outgrown with age. Rather, it is a lifelong disorder that can impact individuals across the lifespan. Below we will we will discuss the impact of ADHD on aging individuals, including how symptoms may change over time and how the diagnosis and treatment of ADHD may differ for older adults.

As individuals with ADHD age, they may experience changes in their symptoms. For example, hyperactivity may decrease, while impulsivity and inattention may become more prominent. In addition, older adults with ADHD may develop coping strategies that help them manage their symptoms. For example, they may have learned to create routines, prioritize tasks, and limit distractions. However, aging can also bring new challenges for individuals with ADHD. For example, memory decline and changes in executive functioning can make it more difficult to manage symptoms, and the stress of life transitions, such as retirement or health issues, can exacerbate symptoms.

The diagnosis and treatment of ADHD in older adults can present unique challenges. First, ADHD is often underdiagnosed in adults, and this can be especially true for older adults who may not have been diagnosed during childhood. Second, older adults may be hesitant to seek diagnosis and treatment due to stigma or concerns about medication side effects. Third, older adults may have other medical conditions or take medications that can interact with ADHD medications, which can complicate treatment.

Despite these challenges, diagnosis and treatment of ADHD in older adults can lead to significant improvements in quality of life. Diagnosis may involve a comprehensive evaluation, including interviews with family members, a review of medical history, and psychological testing. Treatment may include medication, behavioral therapies, and lifestyle changes. However, medication dosages may need to be adjusted for older adults, and non-pharmacological interventions, such as cognitive-behavioral therapy, may be preferred in some cases.

In addition to medical interventions, there are also lifestyle changes that can help manage symptoms of ADHD in aging individuals. For example, regular exercise, a healthy diet, and good sleep hygiene can all contribute to better symptom management. Social support and engagement in meaningful activities can also be beneficial for older adults with ADHD.

In conclusion, ADHD is a lifelong disorder that can impact individuals across the lifespan, including older adults. As individuals with ADHD age, they may experience changes in symptoms and new challenges, but diagnosis and treatment can lead to significant improvements in quality of life. Diagnosis and treatment of ADHD in older adults can present unique challenges, but comprehensive evaluation and individualized treatment plans can help manage symptoms and improve overall well-being. Additionally, lifestyle changes such as regular exercise, healthy eating habits, and social support can also contribute to better symptom management.

The changing presentation of ADHD throughout the lifespan

Attention deficit hyperactivity disorder (ADHD) is typically thought of as a childhood disorder, but it can persist into adulthood and even affect individuals in their later years. As people age, the symptoms and challenges of ADHD may change, and it can become more difficult to recognize and manage the disorder. Below we will we will explore how the presentation of ADHD changes throughout the lifespan.

Childhood ADHD is characterized by symptoms such as hyperactivity, impulsivity, and inattention. Children with ADHD may struggle with academic and social functioning, have difficulty following rules, and act out in inappropriate ways. However, as individuals with ADHD age, their symptoms may become less apparent or present in different ways.

In adolescence and young adulthood, the symptoms of ADHD may shift from hyperactivity and impulsivity to inattention and executive functioning difficulties. Adolescents with ADHD may struggle with time management, organization, and completing tasks, which can impact their academic and professional success. They may also experience difficulties with social interactions, as they may struggle to read social cues or have difficulty controlling their emotions.

As adults with ADHD age, they may experience additional challenges related to the disorder. ADHD can impact executive functioning, which can make it difficult to manage finances, maintain a household, or complete daily tasks. It can also lead to difficulties in the workplace, as individuals with ADHD may struggle with time management, meeting deadlines, and staying organized.

In addition, as individuals with ADHD age, they may experience co-occurring medical conditions that can exacerbate ADHD symptoms or make them more difficult to manage. For example, individuals with ADHD may be at increased risk for developing anxiety or depression, which can worsen their symptoms and impact their quality of life.

As individuals with ADHD enter their later years, the symptoms of the disorder may become even more challenging to manage. Cognitive decline and memory issues can make it difficult to remember tasks or complete them in a timely manner. Individuals with ADHD may also struggle with physical limitations that can impact their ability to stay organized or complete tasks.

Despite the challenges associated with ADHD throughout the lifespan, there are strategies that can be effective for managing the disorder. Medications such as stimulants or non-stimulants can be helpful in reducing symptoms, although they may need to be adjusted as individuals age. Behavioral therapies such as cognitive-behavioral therapy or coaching can also be effective in teaching individuals with ADHD strategies for managing their symptoms.

In addition, lifestyle changes such as regular exercise, a healthy diet, and adequate sleep can also be helpful in managing ADHD symptoms throughout the lifespan. These changes can help improve executive functioning and reduce symptoms such as impulsivity and inattention.

In conclusion, ADHD is a disorder that can impact individuals throughout their lives. While the symptoms and challenges associated with the disorder may change as individuals age, there are strategies that can be effective in managing ADHD symptoms at any age. By understanding the unique challenges associated with ADHD at different stages of life, individuals with the disorder and their loved ones can work together to develop effective management strategies that improve quality of life.

Strategies for managing ADHD in older adults

Attention-deficit/hyperactivity disorder (ADHD) is often thought of as a disorder that affects children and adolescents, but it can also impact adults, including those in later life. As people age, they may experience changes in their ADHD symptoms and may face different challenges in managing the disorder. Below we will we will explore the changing presentation of ADHD throughout the lifespan and discuss strategies for managing ADHD in older adults.

ADHD in Children and Adolescents:

In childhood, ADHD is often characterized by hyperactivity, impulsivity, and inattention. Children may struggle with following directions, sitting still, completing tasks, and staying organized. These symptoms can impact academic performance, social relationships, and family dynamics.

ADHD in Adults:

ADHD can continue into adulthood, and symptoms may change as individuals age. While hyperactivity may decrease in adults with ADHD, they may still struggle with impulsivity and inattention. Adults with ADHD may experience difficulties with time management, organization, and completing tasks, which can impact work and personal life. ADHD in adults can also impact relationships, with a tendency towards disorganization, forgetfulness, and impulsive behavior.

ADHD in Older Adults:

While research on ADHD in older adults is limited, studies suggest that ADHD can persist into later life. Symptoms of hyperactivity and impulsivity may continue to decrease, but inattention may persist or even worsen. Older adults with ADHD may experience additional challenges due to age-related changes in cognitive function, such as memory and processing speed.

Managing ADHD in Older Adults:

Managing ADHD in older adults may require different strategies than those used in younger populations. Here are some strategies that may be helpful for managing ADHD in older adults:

1. Medication Management: Medications are a common treatment for ADHD and can be effective in managing symptoms in older adults. However, older adults may be more sensitive to the side effects of medication, and dosages may need to be adjusted. Working closely with a healthcare provider can ensure proper medication management.

2. Behavioral Therapy: Behavioral therapy, such as cognitive-behavioral therapy, can be helpful in teaching coping skills for managing ADHD symptoms. Therapy can help older adults develop strategies for managing impulsivity, improving organization and time management, and addressing emotional regulation.

3. Support Networks: Support from friends, family, and peers can be helpful in managing ADHD. Joining a support group or seeking out peers who also have ADHD can provide a sense of community and understanding.

4. Lifestyle Changes: Maintaining a healthy lifestyle can also be helpful in managing ADHD. Regular exercise, a healthy diet, and adequate sleep can help improve mood, attention, and overall well-being.

5. Environmental Modifications: Making changes to the environment can help older adults with ADHD manage symptoms. Reducing clutter and noise, simplifying routines, and breaking down tasks into smaller steps can help improve focus and decrease distractibility.

In conclusion, while ADHD is often thought of as a disorder that primarily affects children and adolescents, it can persist into adulthood and impact individuals throughout the lifespan. ADHD in older adults may present with different challenges than those in younger populations, but there are strategies available to help manage symptoms and improve overall well-being. Working closely with healthcare providers, seeking out support, and making lifestyle modifications can all be helpful in managing ADHD in older adults.

The impact of aging on ADHD treatment and support

As people age, their needs and circumstances change, and this is true for those living with ADHD. The symptoms of ADHD can present differently throughout the lifespan and can pose unique challenges as an individual enters their later years. Below we will we will explore the impact of aging on ADHD treatment and support and offer strategies for managing ADHD in older adults.

First, it is important to understand the changing presentation of ADHD throughout the lifespan. Children and adolescents with ADHD tend to exhibit symptoms such as hyperactivity, impulsivity, and inattention, which can result in academic and behavioral difficulties. As individuals transition into adulthood, they may experience changes in their symptoms, such as decreased hyperactivity and an increase in internal restlessness and difficulty with time management. In older adults, the symptoms of ADHD can be similar to those experienced in childhood, including difficulties with executive functioning and memory, as well as a decline in cognitive ability. Additionally, as individuals age, they may be more susceptible to co-occurring conditions such as depression and anxiety, which can complicate ADHD treatment.

When it comes to managing ADHD in older adults, treatment and support must be tailored to the unique needs and circumstances of the individual. This may involve a combination of medication, therapy, and lifestyle changes. One approach to medication management for older adults with ADHD is to start with lower doses and increase gradually to achieve the desired effect while minimizing potential side effects. It is also important to take into account any other medications that the individual is taking, as some medications can interact with ADHD medications.

Therapy can also be a helpful tool for managing ADHD in older adults. Cognitive-behavioral therapy (CBT) has been shown to be effective in helping individuals with ADHD develop strategies for managing their symptoms and improving executive functioning. Family and couples therapy can also be beneficial for older adults with ADHD, as it can help to address interpersonal dynamics and improve communication.

In addition to medication and therapy, lifestyle changes can also be helpful for managing ADHD in older adults. Exercise, for example, has been shown to improve executive functioning and attention. Older adults with ADHD may also benefit from routines and structure, as these can help to manage symptoms of impulsivity and distractibility. Mindfulness and meditation practices can also be helpful for managing ADHD symptoms and improving overall well-being.

Finally, it is important to consider the impact of aging on ADHD treatment and support. As individuals age, they may experience changes in their physical and cognitive abilities, which can impact their ability to manage their ADHD symptoms. Additionally, older adults may face unique challenges related to social isolation, financial difficulties, and health concerns, which can further complicate ADHD management. As such, it is important to consider the individual's overall well-being and tailor treatment and support to their unique needs and circumstances.

In conclusion, managing ADHD in older adults requires a multifaceted approach that takes into account the changing presentation of ADHD throughout the lifespan, the individual's unique needs and circumstances, and the impact of aging on treatment and support. By incorporating medication, therapy, lifestyle changes, and a consideration of the individual's overall well-being, older adults with ADHD can manage their symptoms and improve their quality of life.

Chapter Fifteen

Alternative and Complementary Therapies

Alternative and complementary therapies are a popular topic in the treatment of ADHD. While medications and behavioral therapies are the most widely recognized treatments for ADHD, many individuals with ADHD also seek out alternative and complementary therapies to supplement their traditional treatments.

Alternative and complementary therapies refer to non-medical treatments and interventions that aim to improve ADHD symptoms. These can include a wide range of practices, such as mindfulness meditation, dietary supplements, herbal remedies, and yoga.

One of the most popular alternative therapies for ADHD is mindfulness meditation. Mindfulness meditation involves focusing one's attention on the present moment, and has been shown to improve attention and reduce impulsivity in individuals with ADHD. Mindfulness meditation can be practiced in many different ways, such as sitting quietly and focusing on one's breath, or participating in a guided meditation class.

Dietary supplements and herbal remedies are also commonly used as alternative treatments for ADHD. Supplements like omega-3 fatty acids and iron have been shown to improve ADHD symptoms in some individuals. Herbal remedies like ginkgo biloba and St. John's wort are also sometimes used to manage ADHD symptoms, although their effectiveness is less well-studied.

Exercise and physical activity have been shown to be beneficial for individuals with ADHD. Exercise can help improve attention and reduce hyperactivity, and can be a great way to supplement traditional ADHD treatments. Activities like yoga and tai chi can also be beneficial for ADHD, as they promote relaxation and can help reduce stress and anxiety.

Acupuncture is another alternative therapy that has been studied as a treatment for ADHD. Acupuncture involves inserting thin needles into the skin at specific points on the body, and is thought to stimulate the body's natural healing processes. While some studies have suggested that acupuncture can be helpful for ADHD symptoms, more research is needed to fully understand its effectiveness.

It is important to note that while alternative and complementary therapies can be helpful for some individuals with ADHD, they are not a substitute for traditional treatments like medication and behavioral therapy. It is also important to talk to a healthcare professional before trying any alternative or complementary therapies, as some may interact with other medications or have side effects.

In addition to alternative and complementary therapies, lifestyle changes can also be effective in managing ADHD symptoms. Getting enough sleep, eating a balanced diet, and reducing stress can all help improve ADHD symptoms. Additionally, finding ways to manage and reduce distractions in daily life, such as using organizational tools and minimizing sensory input, can be helpful for individuals with ADHD.

In conclusion, alternative and complementary therapies can be effective in managing ADHD symptoms, but should be used in conjunction with traditional treatments like medication and behavioral therapy. Mindfulness meditation, dietary supplements, herbal remedies, exercise, and acupuncture are all potential alternative treatments for ADHD, but it is important to talk to a healthcare professional before trying any of these therapies. Additionally, making lifestyle changes like getting enough sleep, eating a balanced diet, and reducing stress can be effective in managing ADHD symptoms.

The role of alternative treatments in ADHD management

Attention deficit hyperactivity disorder (ADHD) is a neurodevelopmental disorder that affects both children and adults. Although there are several medications and behavioral therapies that have been proven to be effective in managing ADHD symptoms, some individuals may prefer alternative treatments. Below we will we will explore the role of alternative treatments in ADHD management.

Alternative treatments are generally defined as interventions that fall outside of conventional medical practice. These can include dietary supplements, herbal remedies, and mind-body techniques like yoga and meditation. While there is limited scientific evidence supporting the effectiveness of these treatments for ADHD specifically, many individuals with ADHD have reported positive results.

One commonly used alternative treatment for ADHD is dietary supplements. Some of the most commonly used supplements include omega-3 fatty acids, zinc, and magnesium. Omega-3 fatty acids are essential nutrients found in fish oil and have been shown to improve attention and behavior in children with ADHD. Zinc and magnesium are also important for brain function and have been linked to improved attention and mood in individuals with ADHD.

Herbal remedies are another popular alternative treatment for ADHD. One of the most commonly used herbs is Ginkgo biloba, which is believed to improve cognitive function and memory. However, the scientific evidence for its effectiveness in managing ADHD symptoms is limited.

Mind-body techniques like yoga and meditation may also be helpful in managing ADHD symptoms. These techniques can help improve focus, reduce stress, and promote relaxation. Research has shown that mindfulness meditation can improve attention and reduce impulsivity in adults with ADHD.

While alternative treatments can be helpful for some individuals with ADHD, it is important to approach them with caution. Many dietary supplements and herbal remedies can interact with prescription medications and cause unwanted side effects. In addition, the quality and purity of these products are not regulated by the Food and Drug Administration (FDA), which means that there is a risk of contamination and inconsistency in dosing.

It is also important to note that alternative treatments should not be used as a substitute for evidence-based treatments like medication and behavioral therapy. These treatments have been proven to be effective in managing ADHD symptoms and should be the first line of treatment for most individuals with ADHD.

If you are interested in trying alternative treatments for ADHD, it is important to talk to your healthcare provider first. They can help you weigh the potential benefits and risks of these treatments and provide guidance on how to safely incorporate them into your overall treatment plan.

In conclusion, alternative treatments can be a helpful addition to the overall management of ADHD symptoms. While there is limited scientific evidence supporting their effectiveness, many individuals with ADHD have reported positive results. However, it is important to approach these treatments with caution and not use them as a substitute for evidence-based treatments. If you are considering alternative treatments for ADHD, be sure to talk to your healthcare provider first to ensure that they are safe and effective for you.

Mindfulness, meditation, and other complementary therapies

Mindfulness, meditation, and other complementary therapies have become increasingly popular in recent years as a way to manage symptoms of ADHD. These practices focus on increasing awareness of the present moment, developing a non-judgmental attitude, and improving emotional regulation. While there is still limited research on the effectiveness of these therapies for ADHD specifically, some studies have shown promising results.

One of the main benefits of mindfulness and meditation is that they can help improve attention and focus. These practices involve paying attention to the present moment and training the mind to stay focused on a particular object or sensation. This can help people with ADHD develop the ability to stay focused on tasks and ignore distractions.

Mindfulness and meditation can also be helpful for managing stress and anxiety, which are common co-occurring conditions with ADHD. These practices can help individuals become more aware of their thoughts and emotions and develop skills to regulate them. This can lead to a greater sense of calm and well-being.

Another complementary therapy that has shown promise for ADHD management is yoga. Yoga combines physical postures with deep breathing and meditation, making it a holistic approach to improving mental and physical health. Some studies have shown that yoga can improve attention, executive functioning, and mood in individuals with ADHD.

Acupuncture is another complementary therapy that has been used to manage symptoms of ADHD. Acupuncture involves the insertion of fine needles into specific points on the body to stimulate the body's natural healing processes. While there is limited research on the effectiveness of acupuncture for ADHD, some studies have shown that it can improve attention, behavior, and social functioning.

In addition to these complementary therapies, there are also other lifestyle factors that can help manage symptoms of ADHD. Regular exercise has been shown to improve attention, mood, and overall well-being in individuals with ADHD. Getting enough sleep is also important, as lack of sleep can exacerbate ADHD symptoms. Eating a healthy diet that includes plenty of fruits, vegetables, and lean protein can also help support brain function and improve overall health.

It's important to note that while complementary therapies can be helpful in managing ADHD symptoms, they should not be used as a replacement for medication or other evidence-based treatments. It's important to work with a healthcare professional to develop a comprehensive treatment plan that includes medication, therapy, and any complementary therapies that may be helpful.

In summary, mindfulness, meditation, yoga, acupuncture, exercise, sleep, and nutrition are all complementary therapies that can be helpful for managing symptoms of ADHD. While more research is needed to fully understand their effectiveness for ADHD specifically, these practices can be a helpful addition to a comprehensive treatment plan. It's important to work with a healthcare professional to develop an individualized plan that addresses all aspects of ADHD management.

Evaluating the effectiveness of alternative treatments

Alternative treatments for ADHD, including natural remedies and behavioral therapies, have gained popularity in recent years. While medication remains the primary treatment option for managing ADHD symptoms, many individuals seek alternative treatments as a complementary or standalone approach. However, the effectiveness of alternative treatments for ADHD is a matter of debate among healthcare professionals and researchers.

One of the most popular alternative treatments for ADHD is natural remedies. These remedies include supplements, such as omega-3 fatty acids, zinc, and iron, as well as herbs like ginkgo biloba and St. John's Wort. Proponents of natural remedies argue that they are safer and have fewer side effects than medication, making them an appealing option for individuals who may be wary of traditional medication. However, there is limited scientific evidence to support the effectiveness of natural remedies in managing ADHD symptoms. In some cases, natural remedies can interact with medication, resulting in adverse side effects. Therefore, it is important for individuals to consult with a healthcare professional before using natural remedies as a treatment option for ADHD.

Behavioral therapies, such as cognitive-behavioral therapy (CBT) and neurofeedback, are also alternative treatment options for ADHD. CBT is a form of talk therapy that aims to help individuals with ADHD develop coping strategies to manage their symptoms. It can help individuals identify negative patterns of thinking and behavior and replace them with more positive and adaptive ones. Neurofeedback, on the other hand, involves using technology to measure and provide feedback on brain activity. The individual can then learn to regulate their brainwaves to improve attention and focus. While behavioral therapies have shown promise in improving ADHD symptoms, more research is needed to fully understand their effectiveness.

Mindfulness and meditation are also alternative treatments that have gained attention in recent years. These practices involve focusing on the present moment and developing greater awareness of one's thoughts and emotions. Proponents of mindfulness and meditation argue that they can help individuals with ADHD manage their symptoms by improving attention, reducing impulsivity, and decreasing stress levels. While studies have shown some positive effects of mindfulness and meditation on ADHD symptoms, more research is needed to fully understand their impact.

When considering alternative treatments for ADHD, it is important to approach them with caution and seek guidance from healthcare professionals. While some alternative treatments may provide benefits, others may have limited or no effectiveness and could potentially be harmful. Furthermore, alternative treatments should not be used as a substitute for medication or other evidence-based treatments. It is important to work with a healthcare professional to develop a comprehensive treatment plan that is tailored to the individual's needs.

In conclusion, alternative treatments for ADHD have gained popularity in recent years as individuals seek complementary or standalone approaches to managing their symptoms. While natural remedies, behavioral therapies, and mindfulness practices have shown some promise in improving ADHD symptoms, more research is needed to fully understand their effectiveness. Individuals considering alternative treatments should approach them with caution and seek guidance from healthcare professionals. A comprehensive treatment plan that includes medication and evidence-based therapies may be the most effective approach to managing ADHD symptoms.

Chapter Sixteen

ADHD and Technology

ADHD, or attention deficit hyperactivity disorder, is a neurodevelopmental disorder that affects a person's ability to pay attention, control impulsive behavior, and regulate their level of activity. It can cause difficulties in various areas of life, including work, school, and relationships. However, technology has provided many opportunities to help individuals with ADHD manage their symptoms more effectively. Below we will we will discuss the role of technology in ADHD management, the benefits and drawbacks of using technology, and different types of technology that can be useful for individuals with ADHD.

One of the key benefits of technology in ADHD management is that it can provide structure and organization. Many individuals with ADHD struggle with time management, forgetfulness, and disorganization, which can impact their productivity and ability to complete tasks. Technology tools such as digital calendars, reminders, and to-do lists can help individuals stay on track and avoid missing deadlines. They can also help individuals prioritize tasks and break them down into smaller, more manageable steps. By providing a clear structure, these tools can help reduce stress and increase productivity.

Another benefit of technology in ADHD management is that it can help individuals stay focused and avoid distractions. Individuals with ADHD can have difficulty maintaining attention and may be easily distracted by external stimuli. However, there are several technological tools that can help them stay on task. For example, noise-cancelling headphones can help block out external sounds and create a more conducive environment for concentration. There are also apps and browser extensions that can block distracting websites and limit access to social media during work or study sessions.

However, it's important to note that technology can also have drawbacks when it comes to managing ADHD. For example, it's easy to get distracted by the endless notifications and alerts that come with smartphones and other devices. In addition, relying too heavily on technology can sometimes exacerbate existing problems with attention and distractibility. It's important to use technology as a tool, rather than relying on it completely, in order to avoid becoming overly reliant on it.

There are several different types of technology that can be useful for individuals with ADHD. One of the most common types is wearable technology, such as smartwatches and fitness trackers. These devices can help individuals track their activity levels and monitor their sleep, which can be particularly helpful for individuals with ADHD who may struggle with hyperactivity and sleep difficulties. There are also apps that can help individuals track their mood, which can be useful for identifying patterns and triggers.

Another type of technology that can be useful for individuals with ADHD is assistive technology. This includes tools such as text-to-speech software, which can help individuals with reading difficulties or those who prefer auditory learning. Similarly, speech-to-text software can help individuals who struggle with written expression or have difficulty with typing. Assistive technology can also include devices such as fidget toys, which can help individuals with ADHD channel their excess energy and improve their focus.

In conclusion, technology has the potential to be a valuable tool in managing ADHD. It can provide structure and organization, help individuals stay focused, and offer assistance in various areas such as reading, writing, and sleep. However, it's important to be mindful of the potential drawbacks of technology, such as the risk of distraction and becoming overly reliant on devices. By using technology in a balanced and thoughtful way, individuals with ADHD can leverage its benefits to better manage their symptoms and improve their quality of life.

The role of technology in ADHD management and support

Attention-deficit/hyperactivity disorder (ADHD) is a condition that can greatly impact an individual's daily life, including their ability to focus, organize tasks, and complete work efficiently. In recent years, there has been increasing interest in using technology to help manage and support individuals with ADHD. From apps and online tools to wearable devices and virtual reality, there are many ways that technology is being used to support individuals with ADHD.

One of the most common uses of technology in ADHD management is the use of apps and online tools. These tools can help individuals with ADHD manage their time, stay organized, and improve their focus. For example, apps like Focus@Will and Brain.fm offer specially curated music tracks that can help improve focus and productivity. Other apps like Trello and Todoist offer organizational tools that can help individuals with ADHD manage their daily tasks and keep track of deadlines.

Wearable devices are also being used to support individuals with ADHD. Devices like the Muse headband use EEG technology to monitor brain activity and provide feedback to users on their level of focus and relaxation. This type of feedback can be particularly helpful for individuals with ADHD who may struggle with self-regulation and managing their attention.

Virtual reality is another technology that is being explored as a potential tool for managing ADHD. Researchers are exploring the use of virtual reality environments to help individuals with ADHD improve their attention and cognitive skills. For example, a virtual reality game called Project EVO has been shown to improve attention and cognitive control in individuals with ADHD.

In addition to these technologies, there are also a variety of online support groups and resources available for individuals with ADHD. These resources can provide helpful tips and advice, as well as a community of support for individuals with ADHD and their families.

While technology can be a valuable tool in managing ADHD, it is important to recognize that it is not a substitute for professional treatment. Individuals with ADHD should always consult with a healthcare professional to determine the most appropriate course of treatment for their individual needs.

Moreover, the effectiveness of technology in managing ADHD symptoms varies from person to person. While some individuals may find that technology is helpful in managing their symptoms, others may not find it as effective. It is important for individuals to try different strategies and tools to determine what works best for them.

Another important consideration is the potential for technology to be a distraction for individuals with ADHD. While technology can be a helpful tool, it can also be a source of distraction and can make it more difficult for individuals with ADHD to stay focused. It is important for individuals with ADHD to use technology in a way that is productive and helps them manage their symptoms, rather than as a distraction.

In conclusion, technology has the potential to be a valuable tool in managing and supporting individuals with ADHD. From apps and online tools to wearable devices and virtual reality, there are many ways that technology is being used to support individuals with ADHD. However, it is important to recognize that technology is not a substitute for professional treatment and that its effectiveness varies from person to person. Individuals with ADHD should consult with a healthcare professional to determine the most appropriate course of treatment for their individual needs and should use technology in a way that is productive and helpful.

Assistive devices and apps for organization and productivity

Assistive devices and apps can be incredibly helpful for individuals with ADHD who struggle with organization, time management, and productivity. With the rise of technology, there are now countless options available to help manage ADHD symptoms and make daily life easier.

One popular type of assistive device is a smartwatch or fitness tracker. These devices offer a variety of features that can be helpful for those with ADHD, such as reminders, alarms, and timers. Some models also include fitness tracking features that can help with motivation and goal-setting. By having these reminders and alerts easily accessible on their wrist, individuals with ADHD can better manage their time and stay on track throughout the day.

Another type of assistive device that can be helpful for individuals with ADHD is a digital voice recorder. This can be used to record important information, such as meetings or lectures, that may be difficult to remember later on. By having a recording of the information, individuals with ADHD can review it at their own pace and have a better chance of retaining the information.

In addition to physical devices, there are also numerous apps available that can be helpful for managing ADHD symptoms. For example, there are apps designed specifically for tracking medication schedules and reminders, such as Medisafe or MyTherapy. There are also apps designed to help with organization and productivity, such as Trello or Todoist, which can be used to create to-do lists and set reminders.

Another helpful type of app for individuals with ADHD is a mindfulness or meditation app. These apps offer guided meditations and mindfulness exercises that can help improve focus and reduce stress. Apps like Headspace or Calm are popular options that offer a variety of meditation exercises to choose from.

While assistive devices and apps can be incredibly helpful for managing ADHD symptoms, it's important to note that they are not a replacement for professional treatment. It's still important for individuals with ADHD to work with their healthcare provider to develop a comprehensive treatment plan that may include medication, therapy, and other interventions.

In addition, it's important to choose assistive devices and apps carefully and consider how they will fit into daily life. For example, some individuals with ADHD may find that certain apps are too complex or difficult to use consistently, which can lead to frustration and a lack of effectiveness. It may take some trial and error to find the right combination of devices and apps that work best for each individual.

In conclusion, assistive devices and apps can be incredibly helpful tools for individuals with ADHD who struggle with organization, time management, and productivity. By utilizing these resources, individuals with

ADHD can better manage their symptoms and improve their daily functioning. However, it's important to remember that these devices and apps are not a replacement for professional treatment and should be used in conjunction with a comprehensive treatment plan.

The impact of screen time and digital distractions on ADHD symptoms

The rise of technology has had a significant impact on our lives, including how we manage ADHD. While technology can provide helpful tools and resources for those with ADHD, it can also be a source of distraction and exacerbate symptoms. Below we will we will explore the impact of screen time and digital distractions on ADHD symptoms and what strategies can be used to manage them.

The Relationship between ADHD and Screen Time

Screen time refers to the amount of time spent in front of a screen, including television, computers, and mobile devices. It is no secret that screen time has increased in recent years, with many individuals spending multiple hours each day on devices. This increase in screen time has coincided with a rise in ADHD diagnoses, leading some to speculate that there may be a link between the two.

Studies have shown that excessive screen time can lead to attention problems and hyperactivity, particularly in children. A study published in the Journal of the American Medical Association found that children who spent more than two hours a day watching television or playing video games were more likely to have ADHD symptoms than those who spent less time on screens.

However, it is important to note that while there may be a correlation between screen time and ADHD symptoms, it does not necessarily mean that screen time causes ADHD. Rather, excessive screen time can exacerbate symptoms in those who already have ADHD.

Managing Digital Distractions

For individuals with ADHD, digital distractions can be particularly problematic. The constant notifications, alerts, and endless sources of information can make it difficult to focus and complete tasks. However, there are strategies that can be used to manage digital distractions and improve focus.

One strategy is to use apps or software that limit distractions. For example, apps like Freedom and Cold Turkey can block websites and apps that are known to be distractions during work or study time. Similarly, features like "Do Not Disturb" on mobile devices can silence notifications during designated times.

Another strategy is to establish boundaries around technology use. This may involve setting designated times for checking email or social media, or designating specific times for work or study without distractions. It can also be helpful to establish a technology-free zone, such as the bedroom, to create a clear separation between technology and relaxation.

Mindfulness and meditation can also be helpful in managing digital distractions. Practicing mindfulness can help individuals become more aware of their thoughts and distractions, allowing them to better manage them. Similarly, meditation can help improve focus and attention, making it easier to stay on task and avoid digital distractions.

The Benefits of Technology in ADHD Management

While digital distractions can be a challenge for those with ADHD, technology can also provide many benefits. For example, there are numerous apps and tools designed specifically for individuals with ADHD to help manage symptoms.

One such tool is the Pomodoro Technique, which involves breaking work or study time into 25-minute intervals with five-minute breaks in between. Apps like Focus@Will and Brain.fm provide music designed to improve focus and attention during work or study time. Other apps, like Evernote and Trello, can help with organization and task management.

Telehealth and virtual appointments have also become increasingly popular in ADHD management, allowing individuals to receive treatment and support from the comfort of their own home. This can be particularly helpful for those who struggle with in-person appointments or live in remote areas.

Conclusion

The impact of technology on ADHD management is complex, with both benefits and challenges. Excessive screen time and digital distractions can exacerbate symptoms, but technology can also provide helpful tools and resources for managing ADHD. By implementing strategies to manage digital distractions, individuals with ADHD can better utilize technology for their benefit.

Chapter Seventeen

ADHD and the Media

ADHD, or Attention Deficit Hyperactivity Disorder, is a neurodevelopmental disorder that affects both children and adults. While it is a well-known condition, there are still many misconceptions and stereotypes surrounding ADHD, particularly in the media.

The portrayal of ADHD in the media has often been negative, with many people believing that ADHD is just an excuse for bad behavior or a lack of discipline. This can be harmful to those with ADHD, as it can lead to stigmatization and misunderstandings.

It is important to understand that ADHD is a legitimate medical condition that affects a person's ability to pay attention, focus, and control impulsive behavior. It is caused by differences in brain structure and function and is not a result of poor parenting or a lack of willpower.

Unfortunately, the media has often focused on sensationalized stories about people with ADHD who have gotten into trouble, such as getting in trouble with the law or struggling in school. While these stories are attention-grabbing, they do not accurately represent the experience of most people with ADHD.

In recent years, there has been a push for more accurate representation of ADHD in the media, with more emphasis on the positive aspects of the condition. Many people with ADHD have unique strengths, such as creativity, high energy levels, and the ability to think outside the box. By highlighting these strengths, the media can help reduce stigmatization and promote understanding.

One way that the media can accurately portray ADHD is by sharing stories of people with the condition who have achieved success in their lives. For example, many famous actors, musicians, and entrepreneurs have ADHD, and their stories can be inspiring for others with the condition.

Another way that the media can help promote understanding of ADHD is by providing accurate information about the condition. Many people still have misconceptions about ADHD, such as believing that it is only a childhood condition or that it only affects boys. By providing accurate information, the media can help dispel these myths and provide a more accurate understanding of the condition.

It is also important for the media to highlight the different types of ADHD, as well as the fact that ADHD can co-occur with other conditions, such as anxiety or depression. This can help promote a more nuanced understanding of the condition and ensure that people with ADHD receive appropriate treatment and support.

However, it is also important to recognize that not all media portrayals of ADHD are negative or inaccurate. There are many examples of films, television shows, and books that accurately depict the experiences of people with ADHD and provide a more nuanced understanding of the condition.

For example, the TV show "Parenthood" features a character with ADHD who struggles with organization and impulse control but is also portrayed as creative and empathetic. Similarly, the book "Driven to Distraction" by Edward Hallowell and John Ratey provides a detailed and empathetic look at the experience of ADHD.

In conclusion, the media can play a powerful role in shaping public perception and understanding of ADHD. While there have been many negative and inaccurate portrayals of the condition, there is also a growing movement to provide more accurate and nuanced depictions of ADHD. By highlighting the strengths and achievements of people with ADHD and providing accurate information about the condition, the media can help reduce stigmatization and promote understanding of ADHD.

Representation of ADHD in film, television, and literature

Attention Deficit Hyperactivity Disorder (ADHD) is a neurodevelopmental disorder that affects individuals across the lifespan. It is characterized by inattention, hyperactivity, and impulsivity, which can significantly impact an individual's academic, social, and occupational functioning. While ADHD has been recognized as a legitimate disorder for decades, its representation in the media has been limited and often stigmatizing. Below we will explore the portrayal of ADHD in film, television, and literature and its impact on public perception.

ADHD has been portrayed in various films and television shows, with varying degrees of accuracy and sensitivity. One of the most well-known portrayals of ADHD in film is the character of Dory in Pixar's Finding Nemo and Finding Dory. While Dory's forgetfulness and distractibility are consistent with ADHD symptoms, the portrayal of these symptoms as comical can reinforce stereotypes and trivialize the challenges of living with ADHD. Similarly, the portrayal of the character of Billy in the film Billy Elliot as hyperactive and impulsive can be seen as stigmatizing and perpetuating negative stereotypes.

In contrast, some films and television shows have attempted to portray ADHD in a more accurate and positive light. The character of Max in the film Max Keeble's Big Move is portrayed as intelligent, creative, and capable despite his ADHD symptoms. The television show Parenthood features a character named Max with ADHD, and the show's portrayal of the challenges and strengths of living with ADHD has been praised for its accuracy and sensitivity.

The representation of ADHD in literature has also been mixed. In some cases, ADHD is portrayed as a character flaw or weakness. For example, the character of Bella Swan in the Twilight series is described as being easily distracted and disorganized, which are commonly associated with ADHD symptoms. However, Bella's ADHD-like traits are portrayed as a hindrance to her relationship with Edward, perpetuating the idea that ADHD is a character flaw that needs to be overcome.

In contrast, some authors have portrayed ADHD in a more positive and nuanced way. The novel "The Curious Incident of the Dog in the Night-Time" by Mark Haddon features a protagonist with Asperger's syndrome, but the character's traits are similar to ADHD symptoms. The book has been praised for its realistic portrayal of the challenges and strengths of living with a neurodevelopmental disorder.

The portrayal of ADHD in the media can have a significant impact on public perception and understanding of the disorder. Stigmatizing or inaccurate portrayals can perpetuate negative stereotypes and contribute to misunderstandings about ADHD. However, accurate and sensitive portrayals can increase awareness and understanding of the challenges and strengths of living with ADHD.

In conclusion, the representation of ADHD in film, television, and literature has been mixed. While some portrayals have perpetuated negative stereotypes, others have attempted to portray ADHD in a more accurate and positive light. As awareness and understanding of ADHD continue to grow, it is important that media portrayals of the disorder become more accurate, nuanced, and sensitive to the experiences of individuals with ADHD.

The role of media in raising awareness and reducing stigma

ADHD, or Attention Deficit Hyperactivity Disorder, is a neurological condition that affects millions of people around the world. It is a disorder that primarily impacts attention, hyperactivity, and impulsivity. Despite its prevalence, many people are still unaware of the disorder and its impacts. In recent years, media outlets have played an important role in raising awareness about ADHD and reducing the stigma associated with it. Below we will explore the role of media in raising awareness and reducing stigma surrounding ADHD.

One of the ways in which media has raised awareness about ADHD is through news coverage. News stories can help to educate the public about the disorder and its impacts. They can also provide information about the latest research and treatment options. By sharing real-life stories of individuals with ADHD and their families, news coverage can help to humanize the disorder and increase understanding and empathy for those living with it.

Another way in which media has raised awareness about ADHD is through television shows and movies that feature characters with ADHD. This type of representation can be both positive and negative. On one hand, it can help to destigmatize the disorder by showing that individuals with ADHD are capable of achieving success in their personal and professional lives. On the other hand, it can perpetuate stereotypes and misconceptions about the disorder if the portrayal is inaccurate or overly negative.

In recent years, there have been a number of television shows and movies that have featured characters with ADHD. One notable example is the popular television show, "Parenthood." In this show, Max Braverman, a young boy with ADHD, is a main character. The show portrays Max and his family navigating the challenges of living with ADHD in a realistic and empathetic way. This type of representation can be valuable in raising awareness and reducing stigma.

There are also a number of books and memoirs that have been written by individuals with ADHD. These personal accounts can be powerful tools for raising awareness and reducing stigma. They provide a firsthand account of what it is like to live with ADHD, and can help others to understand the disorder in a more meaningful way. Some examples of books about ADHD include "Driven to Distraction" by Edward Hallowell and John Ratey, and "The ADHD Effect on Marriage" by Melissa Orlov.

While media has played an important role in raising awareness about ADHD, there are also potential downsides to this exposure. For example, media coverage can perpetuate stereotypes and misconceptions about the disorder if it is not accurate or balanced. This can lead to further stigmatization and misunderstanding. Additionally, media exposure can be overwhelming for individuals with ADHD who may struggle with sensory overload and difficulty filtering out distractions.

In conclusion, media has played an important role in raising awareness and reducing stigma surrounding ADHD. News coverage, television shows and movies, and books and memoirs have all contributed to increasing understanding and empathy for individuals with ADHD. However, it is important to be aware of the potential downsides of media exposure and to strive for accurate and balanced representation. By continuing to raise awareness and reduce stigma surrounding ADHD, we can help individuals with the disorder to receive the support and understanding they need to thrive.

Influential documentaries, books, and other resources about ADHD

Attention Deficit Hyperactivity Disorder (ADHD) is a neurodevelopmental disorder that affects both children and adults. The condition is characterized by inattention, hyperactivity, and impulsivity, which can lead to difficulties in academic, social, and occupational settings. While the condition has been known for decades, there has been a growing interest in recent years to raise awareness and reduce stigma surrounding ADHD. One way this has been accomplished is through the creation of documentaries, books, and other resources that provide information and insights into the condition. Below we will we will explore some of the most influential documentaries, books, and resources about ADHD.

One of the most well-known documentaries about ADHD is "ADD & Loving It?!" This documentary was created by Patrick McKenna, a Canadian actor and comedian who was diagnosed with ADHD later in life. In the documentary, McKenna and co-host Rick Green discuss their personal experiences with ADHD and share insights from leading ADHD experts. The documentary covers a range of topics, including the history of ADHD, common symptoms and behaviors, and strategies for managing the condition. The documentary has been widely praised for its informative and engaging approach to the subject matter and has been credited with raising awareness and reducing stigma surrounding ADHD.

Another popular documentary about ADHD is "The Misunderstood Epidemic." This documentary was produced by the National Film Board of Canada and provides a comprehensive look at ADHD in North America. The documentary features interviews with leading experts, as well as people with ADHD and their families. The film covers a range of topics, including the diagnosis and treatment of ADHD, the impact of ADHD on families and communities, and strategies for managing the condition. The documentary has been widely praised for its balanced and informative approach to the subject matter.

In addition to documentaries, there are many books and other resources available about ADHD. One of the most influential books about ADHD is "Driven to Distraction" by Dr. Edward Hallowell and Dr. John Ratey. The book provides a comprehensive overview of ADHD, including its history, symptoms, and diagnosis. The authors also provide practical advice for managing ADHD, including strategies for improving organization and time management. The book has been widely praised for its accessible writing style and helpful tips for managing the condition.

Another influential book about ADHD is "Taking Charge of ADHD" by Dr. Russell Barkley. The book provides a comprehensive overview of ADHD, including its impact on academic and occupational success. The author also provides practical advice for managing ADHD, including strategies for improving organization, time management, and social skills. The book has been widely praised for its helpful tips and strategies for managing the condition.

There are also many online resources available for people with ADHD and their families. One of the most popular resources is ADDitude magazine, which provides information and advice about ADHD. The magazine features articles written by leading ADHD experts, as well as personal stories from people with ADHD and their families. The website also features a range of tools and resources, including a symptom checklist and a directory of ADHD coaches.

Another popular online resource for people with ADHD is CHADD, which stands for Children and Adults with Attention-Deficit/Hyperactivity Disorder. The organization provides information and support to people with ADHD and their families, as well as advocacy for improved treatment options. The website features a range of resources, including articles and webinars, as well as a directory of local support groups.

In conclusion, documentaries, books, and other resources play an important role in raising awareness and reducing stigma surrounding ADHD. They provide valuable information and insights into the condition, as well as practical advice for managing ADHD symptoms. By educating people about ADHD, we can help to improve the lives of those with the condition and reduce the negative impact of stigma and misinformation.

Chapter Eighteen

ADHD Advocacy and Policy

ADHD, or Attention Deficit Hyperactivity Disorder, is a neurodevelopmental disorder that affects millions of people worldwide. Individuals with ADHD often experience difficulties with attention, impulsivity, and hyperactivity, which can impact their daily lives in various ways. As a result, ADHD advocacy and policy have become increasingly important in recent years, with many organizations and individuals working to improve access to resources and support for those with ADHD.

One of the primary goals of ADHD advocacy and policy is to raise awareness about the disorder and reduce stigma surrounding it. Many people with ADHD face discrimination and misunderstandings about their condition, which can make it challenging to access appropriate treatment and support. Advocacy efforts seek to address these issues by providing accurate information about ADHD, highlighting the strengths and challenges of those with the disorder, and promoting acceptance and inclusion.

Another key area of focus for ADHD advocacy and policy is improving access to resources and support for those with the disorder. This includes advocating for increased funding for research, education, and treatment programs, as well as working to improve insurance coverage and access to affordable medications and therapies. Advocates also work to ensure that individuals with ADHD are able to receive appropriate accommodations and support in schools and the workplace, such as extended time on exams, flexible work schedules, or assistive technologies.

Advocacy efforts around ADHD have also been instrumental in promoting the rights and interests of individuals with the disorder. This includes working to eliminate discriminatory practices, such as the denial of employment or educational opportunities based on an ADHD diagnosis. Advocates also work to ensure that individuals with ADHD are included in clinical trials and other research studies, and that their perspectives and experiences are taken into account when developing policies and guidelines related to the disorder.

One notable example of ADHD advocacy and policy in action is the work of the Attention Deficit Disorder Association (ADDA), a nonprofit organization dedicated to providing education, resources, and support for individuals with ADHD. The ADDA advocates for policy changes that improve access to treatment and accommodations for those with ADHD, and also provides a range of programs and services, such as support groups, educational webinars, and a helpline for individuals seeking information and guidance related to ADHD.

Another notable advocacy effort is the CHADD (Children and Adults with Attention-Deficit/Hyperactivity Disorder) organization, which works to improve the lives of individuals with ADHD through advocacy, education, and support. The organization advocates for policy changes that improve access to care and services, and also provides a range of resources for individuals with ADHD and their families, including information on treatment options, education and employment accommodations, and support groups.

Overall, ADHD advocacy and policy play an essential role in promoting the rights and well-being of individuals with ADHD. By raising awareness, improving access to resources and support, and advocating for policy changes, these efforts help to reduce stigma, improve treatment options, and empower individuals with ADHD to live fulfilling and productive lives.

The importance of ADHD advocacy and policy change

Attention Deficit Hyperactivity Disorder (ADHD) is a neurodevelopmental disorder that affects people of all ages. It is a condition that impacts various aspects of life, including education, employment, relationships, and mental health. Therefore, it is essential to have effective policies and advocacy to ensure that people with ADHD receive the appropriate care and support they need to succeed.

ADHD advocacy refers to the efforts to raise awareness and promote change in policies and laws to benefit people with ADHD. Policy change is crucial to ensuring that people with ADHD receive equal treatment and are not discriminated against in various areas of life. ADHD advocacy can take various forms, such as lobbying for laws and regulations, creating awareness through public campaigns, and promoting research to better understand ADHD.

One of the primary reasons for ADHD advocacy is to increase awareness and understanding of the disorder. Many people misunderstand ADHD and associate it with laziness or lack of discipline, which can lead to stigmatization and discrimination. However, ADHD is a neurodevelopmental disorder that affects the brain's ability to regulate attention, impulsivity, and hyperactivity. Therefore, ADHD advocacy is necessary to create a better understanding of the disorder and reduce the stigma that people with ADHD may face.

Another critical area of ADHD advocacy is education. Effective policies are necessary to ensure that children with ADHD receive appropriate education and support. For example, accommodations such as extra time for assignments and tests, preferential seating, and assistive technology can make a significant difference in the academic success of students with ADHD. It is also essential to provide teachers and school staff with training on how to recognize and support students with ADHD.

In the workplace, policies that provide reasonable accommodations and support for employees with ADHD are essential. Accommodations such as flexible schedules, clear communication, and task modification can help employees with ADHD manage their symptoms and perform their jobs effectively. Advocacy for such policies can help reduce discrimination against employees with ADHD and promote equal employment opportunities.

ADHD advocacy is also essential for mental health. Many people with ADHD also experience co-occurring mental health conditions such as anxiety and depression. Effective policies and advocacy can ensure that people with ADHD receive appropriate mental health care and support. Policies that promote access to mental health services and support groups can also help people with ADHD and their families cope with the challenges that come with the disorder.

ADHD advocacy also plays a crucial role in promoting research on the disorder. Research can help improve our understanding of ADHD and lead to better treatments and support for people with the disorder. Therefore, advocacy for funding and support for ADHD research is essential.

In conclusion, ADHD advocacy and policy change are crucial for ensuring that people with ADHD receive the appropriate care and support they need to succeed. Advocacy efforts can help increase awareness and understanding of the disorder, promote effective education and employment policies, and provide access to mental health care and support. Advocacy can also promote research on the disorder, leading to better treatments and support for people with ADHD. It is essential to continue advocacy efforts to improve the lives of people with ADHD and reduce the stigma associated with the disorder.

Understanding disability rights and legislation

Attention Deficit Hyperactivity Disorder (ADHD) is a condition that affects millions of individuals worldwide. In the United States, around 10% of children have been diagnosed with ADHD, and about 4% of adults are affected. While ADHD is recognized as a disability, it is often misunderstood or overlooked. However, understanding disability rights and legislation can help individuals with ADHD get the support and accommodations they need to succeed in school and the workplace.

The Americans with Disabilities Act (ADA) is a federal law that prohibits discrimination against individuals with disabilities in all aspects of life. This includes employment, education, housing, and public accommodations. ADHD is considered a disability under the ADA, and individuals with ADHD are entitled to protection under this law.

The ADA defines a disability as a physical or mental impairment that substantially limits one or more major life activities. Major life activities include things like caring for oneself, learning, speaking, and working. For individuals with ADHD, their impairment may substantially limit their ability to focus, remember information, and complete tasks in a timely manner. These limitations can affect their ability to learn, work, and care for themselves.

Under the ADA, employers and schools are required to provide reasonable accommodations for individuals with disabilities. Reasonable accommodations are changes or adjustments to a job, class, or environment that allow an individual with a disability to perform essential functions of the job or participate fully in educational activities. Examples of reasonable accommodations for individuals with ADHD include extended time on tests, access to a quiet work or study space, and the use of assistive technology.

Individuals with ADHD must disclose their disability to their employer or school in order to receive accommodations. However, disclosure can be a difficult decision. While the ADA prohibits discrimination against individuals with disabilities, stigma and misconceptions about ADHD can still exist. Some individuals may fear that disclosing their ADHD will result in negative consequences, such as being passed over for promotions or being stigmatized by peers.

In addition to the ADA, there are other laws and policies that affect individuals with ADHD. The Individuals with Disabilities Education Act (IDEA) is a federal law that ensures that children with disabilities receive appropriate educational services and supports. Under IDEA, children with ADHD may be eligible for an Individualized Education Plan (IEP) or a 504 plan, which outlines the accommodations and services they need to succeed in school.

There are also state-level disability laws and policies that can affect individuals with ADHD. For example, some states have laws that require employers to provide accommodations for individuals with disabilities, while others have laws that require schools to screen students for ADHD.

Advocacy and policy change are critical for ensuring that individuals with ADHD receive the support and accommodations they need to succeed. ADHD advocacy organizations work to raise awareness about ADHD, promote research into the condition, and advocate for policies and legislation that support individuals with ADHD. Some examples of ADHD advocacy organizations include CHADD (Children and Adults with Attention-Deficit/Hyperactivity Disorder), the Attention Deficit Disorder Association (ADDA), and the National Institute of Mental Health (NIMH).

In addition to advocacy organizations, individuals with ADHD can also advocate for themselves by speaking up about their needs and experiences. This can involve disclosing their ADHD to their employer or school, advocating for reasonable accommodations, and sharing their story with others to raise awareness and reduce stigma.

In conclusion, understanding disability rights and legislation is critical for individuals with ADHD to receive the support and accommodations they need to succeed in school and the workplace. The ADA, IDEA, and state-level disability laws provide protections and guidelines for individuals with disabilities, including those with ADHD. Advocacy organizations and self-advocacy are also important tools for promoting awareness and policy change. By working together, individuals with ADHD and their supporters can ensure that everyone has equal opportunities to reach their full potential.

Getting involved in advocacy and policy initiatives

Attention Deficit Hyperactivity Disorder (ADHD) is a complex neurodevelopmental disorder that affects individuals of all ages. Although there is no known cure for ADHD, early diagnosis and effective management can lead to improved outcomes for individuals living with this condition. In addition to medical treatment and therapy, advocacy and policy initiatives are important for individuals with ADHD to access appropriate support and accommodations. Below we will we will explore the importance of ADHD advocacy and policy initiatives, including understanding disability rights and legislation, and how individuals can get involved in advocating for themselves and others with ADHD.

The importance of ADHD advocacy and policy initiatives cannot be overstated. Without these efforts, individuals with ADHD may struggle to access appropriate support and accommodations in various areas of life, including education, employment, and healthcare. Advocacy efforts can help raise awareness about ADHD and promote understanding and acceptance of individuals with this condition. Additionally, advocacy efforts can promote changes in policy and legislation that better support individuals with ADHD.

One critical aspect of ADHD advocacy and policy initiatives is understanding disability rights and legislation. The Americans with Disabilities Act (ADA) is a federal law that prohibits discrimination against individuals with disabilities, including ADHD, in various areas of life. The ADA ensures that individuals with disabilities have equal opportunities in areas such as employment, education, transportation, and healthcare. The ADA also requires that reasonable accommodations be made to ensure equal access for individuals with disabilities. For example, in an educational setting, reasonable accommodations may include extra time on tests or the ability to take tests in a quiet environment.

In addition to the ADA, there are other laws and regulations that protect the rights of individuals with disabilities. The Individuals with Disabilities Education Act (IDEA) ensures that students with disabilities receive appropriate educational services and supports, including special education and related services. Section 504 of the Rehabilitation Act of 1973 prohibits discrimination based on disability in programs and activities that receive federal funding, including public schools.

Understanding disability rights and legislation is essential for individuals with ADHD to access appropriate support and accommodations. However, it is equally important for individuals with ADHD to get involved in advocacy and policy initiatives. One way to get involved is by joining a local or national advocacy group. For example, CHADD (Children and Adults with Attention-Deficit/Hyperactivity Disorder) is a national nonprofit organization that provides support, education, and advocacy for individuals with ADHD and their families. The ADHD Coaches Organization (ACO) is another national organization that provides coaching services and resources for individuals with ADHD.

Individuals with ADHD can also advocate for themselves by learning about their legal rights and advocating for appropriate accommodations. This may involve working with healthcare providers, educators, and employers to ensure that necessary accommodations are made. For example, in a workplace setting, individuals with ADHD may request accommodations such as flexible work hours, a quiet workspace, or the ability to take breaks when needed.

In addition to advocating for themselves, individuals with ADHD can also advocate for policy change at the local, state, or national level. This may involve contacting elected officials, participating in public hearings, or sharing personal stories about the impact of ADHD on their lives. Advocacy efforts can also involve collaborating with other organizations or groups that support individuals with disabilities.

In conclusion, ADHD advocacy and policy initiatives are critical for individuals with ADHD to access appropriate support and accommodations in various areas of life. Understanding disability rights and legislation is essential for individuals with ADHD to ensure that they receive the necessary accommodations and services. Additionally, getting involved in advocacy and policy initiatives can help raise awareness about ADHD and promote policy changes that better support individuals with this condition. Individuals with ADHD can get involved in advocacy efforts by joining advocacy groups, advocating for themselves, and advocating for policy change at the local, state, or national level. By working together to promote ADHD advocacy and policy initiatives, we can improve outcomes

Chapter Nineteen

ADHD Research and Future Directions

Attention-deficit/hyperactivity disorder (ADHD) is a neurodevelopmental disorder that affects both children and adults. ADHD is characterized by symptoms such as inattention, hyperactivity, and impulsivity, which can significantly impact a person's ability to function in daily life. While there are currently effective treatments for ADHD, there is still much to learn about this disorder, and ongoing research is essential for improving diagnosis, treatment, and management.

ADHD research has made significant strides in recent years, but there is still much to be done. Here are some of the latest developments and future directions in ADHD research:

1. Genetics: While it is widely believed that genetics play a significant role in the development of ADHD, the specific genes involved are still being identified. Recent studies have identified specific genetic variants that are associated with ADHD, but much more research is needed to understand the complex interplay between genetics and environmental factors in the development of ADHD.

2. Brain Imaging: Brain imaging studies have revealed differences in brain structure and function between individuals with ADHD and those without. These studies have helped to increase our understanding of the neurological underpinnings of ADHD and may lead to more effective treatments in the future.

3. Environmental Factors: While genetics play a significant role in the development of ADHD, environmental factors such as prenatal exposure to toxins and childhood trauma may also contribute to the disorder. More research is needed to understand the impact of these environmental factors on the development of ADHD and how they can be mitigated.

4. Medication: While medications such as stimulants and non-stimulants are effective in managing ADHD symptoms, they do not work for everyone, and there are side effects to consider. Ongoing research is focused on developing new medications that may be more effective and have fewer side effects.

5. Non-Pharmacological Interventions: In addition to medication, non-pharmacological interventions such as behavioral therapy, cognitive-behavioral therapy, and mindfulness-based interventions have been shown to be effective in managing ADHD symptoms. Ongoing research is focused on developing and refining these interventions to improve outcomes for individuals with ADHD.

6. Comorbidities: ADHD often co-occurs with other mental health disorders, such as anxiety and depression. Ongoing research is focused on understanding the relationship between ADHD and comorbidities, as well as developing effective treatment approaches that address both conditions.

7. Lifespan: ADHD is typically diagnosed in childhood, but symptoms often persist into adulthood. Ongoing research is focused on understanding how ADHD symptoms change over the lifespan, as well as developing effective treatment approaches for adults with ADHD.

The future of ADHD research is promising, with ongoing studies focused on improving our understanding of the disorder and developing more effective treatments. However, there are also significant challenges in ADHD research, including the need for large-scale studies with diverse populations, funding limitations, and the difficulty of objectively measuring ADHD symptoms. Nonetheless, with continued investment in research, we can improve outcomes for individuals with ADHD and their families.

Current trends and findings in ADHD research

ADHD is a neurodevelopmental disorder that affects individuals across the lifespan. Over the years, numerous studies have been conducted to better understand ADHD, its causes, and effective treatment approaches. Below we will explore some of the current trends and findings in ADHD research.

One significant finding in ADHD research is the understanding of the brain regions and networks involved in the disorder. Researchers have identified differences in the brains of individuals with ADHD compared to those without the disorder, including differences in the prefrontal cortex, the basal ganglia, and the cerebellum. The prefrontal cortex, which is responsible for executive functions such as working memory and attention, has been found to be smaller in individuals with ADHD. The basal ganglia, which is involved in regulating movements, has also been found to be less active in individuals with ADHD. Finally, the cerebellum, which is involved in motor control and coordination, has been found to be abnormal in individuals with ADHD.

Another important area of ADHD research is the investigation of genetic and environmental factors that may contribute to the disorder. It is widely accepted that ADHD has a genetic component, with research suggesting that up to 80% of the risk for ADHD is inherited. However, environmental factors such as prenatal exposure to alcohol or smoking, low birth weight, and premature birth have also been linked to an increased risk for developing ADHD. Research is ongoing to identify specific genes and environmental factors that contribute to ADHD, as well as to understand how they interact with each other.

In terms of treatment, there is growing evidence for the effectiveness of behavioral interventions for individuals with ADHD. Behavioral interventions, such as parent training, behavioral therapy, and school-based interventions, have been shown to improve ADHD symptoms and functioning. Additionally, medication remains a cornerstone of ADHD treatment, with stimulant medications being the most commonly prescribed medication for the disorder. However, research is ongoing to develop new medications and treatment approaches that may be more effective or have fewer side effects.

Finally, there is a growing emphasis on the importance of understanding the impact of ADHD on individuals across the lifespan. While ADHD is often thought of as a disorder of childhood, it can persist into adulthood and has been linked to numerous negative outcomes, including lower educational and occupational attainment, lower income, and increased risk for substance use disorders. Research is increasingly focused on understanding the long-term outcomes of individuals with ADHD and developing interventions to improve these outcomes.

Overall, ADHD research is a rapidly evolving field that has made significant strides in recent years. From identifying brain differences to understanding the genetic and environmental factors that contribute to the disorder, to developing effective interventions and understanding the impact of ADHD across the lifespan, researchers are making progress in better understanding ADHD and how to effectively treat and manage it.

The role of neuroscience in understanding ADHD

The study of neuroscience has provided valuable insight into the underlying mechanisms and neural pathways involved in attention-deficit/hyperactivity disorder (ADHD). ADHD is a neurodevelopmental disorder characterized by symptoms of inattention, hyperactivity, and impulsivity that can significantly impact daily functioning. In recent years, researchers have used various neuroimaging techniques to explore the structural and functional differences in the brains of individuals with ADHD compared to those without. Below we will discuss the role of neuroscience in understanding ADHD.

One of the most significant findings from neuroscience research is the presence of structural differences in the brains of individuals with ADHD. Studies have consistently shown that the prefrontal cortex, which is responsible for executive functioning such as decision-making, planning, and impulse control, is smaller in individuals with ADHD. The basal ganglia, which plays a role in motor control and reward processing, is also smaller in those with the disorder. These findings suggest that the abnormalities in the prefrontal cortex and basal ganglia may contribute to the behavioral symptoms of ADHD.

Furthermore, functional magnetic resonance imaging (fMRI) studies have revealed differences in brain activity between individuals with ADHD and those without. For example, one study found that individuals with ADHD have reduced activation in the prefrontal cortex during tasks that require attention and cognitive control. Another study found that individuals with ADHD have increased activation in the basal ganglia during tasks that involve reward processing. These findings provide evidence for the neural mechanisms underlying the symptoms of ADHD.

Neuroscience research has also helped to shed light on the genetic factors that contribute to ADHD. Twin studies have shown that genetics play a significant role in the development of the disorder, with heritability estimated to be around 70-80%. Genome-wide association studies have identified several genetic variants associated with ADHD, including those involved in the regulation of dopamine signaling, a neurotransmitter that plays a crucial role in reward processing and motivation.

In addition to understanding the biological mechanisms of ADHD, neuroscience research has also contributed to the development of new treatments for the disorder. For example, neurofeedback, a technique that uses real-time feedback on brain activity to train individuals to regulate their brain function, has shown promise in reducing symptoms of ADHD. fMRI studies have shown that neurofeedback can increase activity in the prefrontal cortex and reduce activity in the default mode network, a network of brain regions associated with mind-wandering and inattention.

Overall, the role of neuroscience in understanding ADHD has been crucial in providing insight into the biological mechanisms of the disorder. The use of neuroimaging techniques has revealed structural and functional differences in the brains of individuals with ADHD, while genetic studies have identified several genetic variants associated with the disorder. This knowledge has also led to the development of new treatments for ADHD, such as neurofeedback. Continued research in the field of neuroscience is essential for further understanding the disorder and developing more effective interventions.

Future directions and potential breakthroughs in ADHD treatment

Attention Deficit Hyperactivity Disorder (ADHD) is a neurodevelopmental disorder that affects approximately 5-10% of children and 2-5% of adults worldwide. While there are several treatment options available for ADHD, researchers are still exploring new ways to improve the lives of those affected by this disorder. Below we will discuss some of the latest research and potential breakthroughs in ADHD treatment.

One area of research that has gained significant attention in recent years is neuroimaging. Neuroimaging techniques allow researchers to study the brain structure and activity of individuals with ADHD. By using techniques such as functional magnetic resonance imaging (fMRI), researchers have been able to identify differences in the brain activity of individuals with ADHD compared to those without. For example, studies have shown that individuals with ADHD have reduced activity in the prefrontal cortex, a brain region responsible for executive function, attention, and decision-making.

The use of neuroimaging techniques has also led to the development of new treatment options. One promising therapy is neurofeedback, which involves training individuals to regulate their brain activity using real-time feedback from neuroimaging. Several studies have shown that neurofeedback can improve attention and reduce symptoms of ADHD in both children and adults. While more research is needed to determine the long-term effectiveness of neurofeedback, it holds promise as a non-invasive and drug-free treatment option.

Another area of research that has shown promise in ADHD treatment is genetics. Studies have identified several genes that may be associated with an increased risk of developing ADHD. Researchers are now exploring the potential of gene therapy, which involves altering the expression of genes associated with ADHD to reduce symptoms. While gene therapy is still in the early stages of development, it holds the potential to provide long-term relief for individuals with ADHD.

In addition to neuroimaging and genetics, researchers are also exploring the potential of new medication options. While stimulant medications such as Ritalin and Adderall have been the primary treatment option for ADHD for several decades, they are not effective for everyone and can have side effects. Researchers are now exploring the potential of new medications that target different neurotransmitters in the brain. For example, a new medication called viloxazine has been shown to improve symptoms of ADHD by targeting the norepinephrine system in the brain. While more research is needed, viloxazine and other non-stimulant medications hold promise as alternative treatment options.

Along with these new treatment options, researchers are also exploring the potential of lifestyle interventions. Studies have shown that exercise, a healthy diet, and regular sleep can improve symptoms of ADHD. Additionally, mindfulness meditation and cognitive-behavioral therapy have been shown to be effective in reducing symptoms and improving quality of life for individuals with ADHD.

Looking forward, researchers are also exploring the potential of digital health technologies in ADHD treatment. Smartphone apps and wearable devices have the potential to provide real-time feedback and support for individuals with ADHD. For example, an app called "Focus@Will" uses music to improve focus and concentration, while another app called "CogCubed" measures attention and provides feedback to users. While more research is needed to determine the effectiveness of these technologies, they hold promise as convenient and accessible treatment options.

In conclusion, researchers are making significant strides in understanding ADHD and developing new treatment options. Advances in neuroimaging, genetics, medication, lifestyle interventions, and digital health technologies all hold promise in improving the lives of those with ADHD. While there is still much to be learned about this disorder, these breakthroughs provide hope for a brighter future for individuals with ADHD and their families.

Chapter Twenty

Staying Informed and Connected

Staying informed and connected is essential for individuals with ADHD who are seeking to manage their condition effectively. There is a wealth of information available on ADHD, and keeping up with the latest research, treatment options, and support resources can be extremely helpful. Below we will explore some ways in which individuals with ADHD can stay informed and connected to the latest developments in the field.

One of the best ways to stay informed about ADHD is to keep up with the latest research. The scientific understanding of ADHD is constantly evolving, and keeping up with the latest findings can be extremely helpful in managing the condition. Many online resources provide access to the latest research, including academic journals, medical publications, and other scientific sources. Individuals with ADHD can also attend conferences and events that focus on the condition, which provide an opportunity to hear from experts in the field and to connect with others who are dealing with similar challenges.

In addition to research and scientific publications, there are also many support groups and online communities that individuals with ADHD can join. These groups can provide a wealth of information and support, and can be a great way to connect with others who are dealing with similar challenges. Many of these groups provide access to experts in the field, as well as to other individuals with ADHD who have found ways to manage their condition effectively. Joining an online community or support group can also be a great way to stay motivated and focused on managing the condition.

Another way to stay informed and connected is to work with a healthcare professional who specializes in ADHD. Many doctors, therapists, and other healthcare providers have extensive experience working with individuals with ADHD, and can provide valuable guidance and support. They can also provide access to the latest treatment options, including medications, therapy, and other interventions that can help manage symptoms and improve overall functioning.

Finally, it's important to stay informed about the latest technological advancements that can help manage ADHD. Many apps, tools, and other resources have been developed specifically for individuals with ADHD, and can be extremely helpful in managing symptoms and improving daily functioning. These tools can include everything from organizational apps to meditation and mindfulness apps to specialized software that can help with tasks like time management and project planning.

In conclusion, staying informed and connected is essential for individuals with ADHD who are seeking to manage their condition effectively. By keeping up with the latest research, joining support groups and online communities, working with healthcare professionals who specialize in ADHD, and staying informed about the latest technological advancements, individuals with ADHD can stay motivated and focused on managing their symptoms and improving their daily functioning. With the right resources and support, it's possible to live a fulfilling and successful life with ADHD.

Keeping up-to-date with ADHD research and news

Keeping up-to-date with ADHD research and news is crucial for individuals with ADHD, their families, and healthcare professionals. With new studies and advancements in research, there are constantly changing perspectives and treatments for ADHD. It is essential to stay informed to make informed decisions and take necessary actions. Below we will discuss the importance of keeping up-to-date with ADHD research and news and ways to stay connected.

ADHD is a complex neurodevelopmental disorder that affects people of all ages. It is characterized by symptoms of inattention, hyperactivity, and impulsivity that affect everyday life, including academic and social functioning. Research has come a long way in understanding the causes and symptoms of ADHD, which has led to the development of effective treatments. However, there is still much to learn about ADHD, and new research and developments are continually emerging.

One of the main reasons to stay up-to-date with ADHD research and news is to be informed about new treatments and interventions. For example, recent studies have shown that mindfulness-based interventions can be effective in reducing ADHD symptoms. Keeping up-to-date with research can inform individuals with ADHD and their families about new treatment options and interventions that can improve their quality of life.

Another reason to stay informed is to be aware of new findings on the causes and underlying mechanisms of ADHD. With advancements in neuroscience, there is a better understanding of the neurobiology of ADHD, including the role of dopamine and other neurotransmitters. Keeping up-to-date with research in this area can inform healthcare professionals and individuals with ADHD about new treatments and interventions based on these findings.

In addition, staying informed about ADHD research and news can help reduce stigma and raise awareness of the disorder. ADHD is still widely misunderstood and stigmatized, and staying informed can help educate others and promote understanding. With accurate and up-to-date information, individuals with ADHD and their families can advocate for themselves and raise awareness about the challenges of living with ADHD.

There are many ways to stay up-to-date with ADHD research and news. One of the easiest ways is to follow reputable sources online, such as the National Institute of Mental Health (NIMH), the Centers for Disease Control and Prevention (CDC), and the Attention Deficit Disorder Association (ADDA). These organizations provide up-to-date information on research, news, and resources for individuals with ADHD and their families.

Another way to stay informed is to attend conferences and events focused on ADHD. These events bring together healthcare professionals, researchers, and individuals with ADHD and their families to share information, research, and best practices. Attending these events can provide valuable information and resources and help individuals with ADHD and their families connect with others in the ADHD community.

Additionally, joining support groups or online communities can provide a wealth of information and support for individuals with ADHD and their families. These groups can provide a safe and supportive space to share experiences, ask questions, and learn about the latest research and treatments.

In conclusion, staying up-to-date with ADHD research and news is essential for individuals with ADHD, their families, and healthcare professionals. It is crucial to stay informed about new treatments, interventions, and research findings to make informed decisions and take necessary actions.

Additionally, staying informed can help reduce stigma, raise awareness, and promote understanding of ADHD. There are many ways to stay connected, including following reputable sources online, attending conferences and events, and joining support groups or online communities. By staying informed, individuals with ADHD and their families can lead fulfilling and successful lives.

The role of conferences, seminars, and workshops

The field of ADHD research and treatment is constantly evolving, and it can be challenging to stay up-to-date with the latest developments. Conferences, seminars, and workshops can provide valuable opportunities for individuals to learn about current research, treatment options, and strategies for managing ADHD symptoms.

One of the key benefits of attending conferences, seminars, and workshops is the opportunity to hear directly from experts in the field. Many events feature presentations from leading researchers, clinicians, and advocates, who can share the latest findings and insights about ADHD. These presentations can help attendees to better understand the science behind ADHD, as well as the most effective approaches for treatment and management.

In addition to formal presentations, conferences, seminars, and workshops often provide opportunities for networking and information-sharing. Attendees can connect with others who have ADHD, as well as with professionals and advocates who are dedicated to improving the lives of people with ADHD. This can be particularly valuable for individuals who feel isolated or uncertain about how to manage their symptoms.

Another benefit of attending these events is the opportunity to learn about new treatment options and strategies for managing ADHD symptoms. Many conferences and workshops feature sessions on topics such as medication management, behavioral therapy, and lifestyle changes that can help individuals with ADHD to better manage their symptoms. By attending these events, individuals can gain practical tools and insights that can help them to improve their daily lives.

Conferences, seminars, and workshops can also provide a platform for advocacy and policy change. Many events feature sessions focused on the latest research and policy initiatives related to ADHD, as well as opportunities to meet with legislators and other policymakers. By attending these events and becoming involved in advocacy efforts, individuals with ADHD can help to shape the conversation about ADHD research, treatment, and policy.

For individuals who are unable to attend conferences, seminars, and workshops in person, many events offer online options such as live streaming or recorded sessions. These options can provide an accessible way for individuals to stay informed about the latest developments in the field of ADHD.

In addition to attending events, individuals can also stay informed about ADHD research and news by subscribing to newsletters, blogs, and other resources focused on ADHD. There are many websites, podcasts, and social media accounts dedicated to sharing information about ADHD, and subscribing to these resources can provide a steady stream of information and insights.

Overall, staying informed and connected is an important part of managing ADHD. Conferences, seminars, and workshops can provide valuable opportunities for individuals to learn about current research, treatment options, and strategies for managing symptoms. By attending these events and staying connected with other individuals with ADHD and professionals in the field, individuals can gain the tools and support they need to live well with ADHD.

Tips for staying informed and connected within the ADHD community

Attention Deficit Hyperactivity Disorder (ADHD) can have a significant impact on a person's life, and it is essential to stay informed and connected within the ADHD community to manage the condition effectively. Below we will we will discuss some tips for staying informed and connected within the ADHD community.

Join a support group

Joining an ADHD support group can help you connect with others who understand what you are going through. Support groups can provide a safe space for you to share your experiences and learn from others. You can find local support groups through your doctor, therapist, or online. Many online support groups have chat rooms, forums, and virtual meetings that allow you to connect with others from the comfort of your own home.

Attend conferences, seminars, and workshops

Attending conferences, seminars, and workshops can provide you with valuable information about the latest research and treatments for ADHD. These events can also be an excellent opportunity to connect with others who are interested in ADHD. Many conferences and workshops offer breakout sessions and networking opportunities that allow you to connect with others who share your interests.

Use social media to connect with others

Social media can be a powerful tool for connecting with others who have ADHD. You can follow ADHD organizations, support groups, and advocates on social media platforms like Facebook, Twitter, and Instagram. These organizations often post articles, tips, and resources that can help you stay informed and connected.

Read books and articles about ADHD

Reading books and articles about ADHD can provide you with valuable information and insights into the condition. You can find books and articles on a wide range of topics, including the latest research, treatment options, and coping strategies. You can also find personal stories from people who have ADHD, which can help you feel less alone.

Educate yourself about your condition

One of the best ways to stay informed about ADHD is to educate yourself about the condition. Learn as much as you can about the symptoms, causes, and treatments for ADHD. Talk to your doctor, therapist, or other healthcare professionals about the condition and ask questions. Being informed about your condition can help you make informed decisions about your treatment and manage your symptoms effectively.

Volunteer with ADHD organizations

Volunteering with ADHD organizations can be an excellent way to connect with others who share your interests and help make a difference in the lives of people with ADHD. Many organizations rely on volunteers to help with events, fundraising, and advocacy efforts. Volunteering can also provide you with opportunities to learn new skills and gain valuable experience.

In conclusion, staying informed and connected within the ADHD community is essential for managing the condition effectively. Joining a support group, attending conferences, using social media, reading books and articles, educating yourself, and volunteering are all great ways to stay informed and connected. By staying informed and connected, you can learn from others, stay up-to-date on the latest research and treatments, and find the support you need to manage your ADHD effectively.

Chapter Twenty-One

Personal Stories and Experiences

Personal stories and experiences can be incredibly powerful in providing insight and understanding about a particular topic. When it comes to ADHD, there are countless stories of individuals who have lived with this condition and the various ways it has affected their lives.

One of the most important aspects of personal stories and experiences is that they can help reduce stigma and increase understanding about ADHD. Often, the public perception of ADHD is limited to stereotypes of hyperactive children who can't sit still or pay attention in class. However, personal stories can show that ADHD is much more complex than this and can affect individuals of all ages and backgrounds.

Furthermore, personal stories can provide a sense of validation and connection for those who are living with ADHD. It can be isolating to feel like you're the only one experiencing the challenges that come with ADHD, but hearing from others who have gone through similar struggles can provide a sense of community and support.

In recent years, there has been a growing movement of individuals sharing their personal experiences with ADHD through various mediums such as blogs, podcasts, and social media. These platforms allow for individuals to connect with others who are going through similar experiences and provide a platform for sharing their stories.

One example of this is the popular podcast "The ADHD Effect on Marriage" hosted by Melissa Orlov, which explores the impact of ADHD on relationships. Orlov uses personal stories from her own experience as well as those of her guests to provide insight and guidance for individuals navigating the challenges of ADHD in their relationships.

Personal stories can also be a valuable tool in raising awareness and advocating for policy change. For example, the "Dear ADHD" campaign, started by ADHD advocate Rene Brooks, encourages individuals to write letters to their ADHD sharing their personal experiences with the condition. These letters are then compiled and shared on social media to raise awareness and advocate for change.

It's important to note that while personal stories can be incredibly powerful, they are not a substitute for scientific research and evidence-based treatment. However, personal stories can provide context and nuance to research findings and can help researchers and healthcare professionals better understand the lived experiences of those with ADHD.

In addition, personal stories can also provide insights into alternative and complementary treatments for ADHD. For example, individuals may share their experiences with non-traditional treatments such as meditation or exercise, which can provide valuable information for others seeking alternative methods of managing their ADHD symptoms.

It's also important to recognize that sharing personal stories can be a vulnerable experience, and not everyone may feel comfortable doing so. However, for those who do choose to share their stories, it can be a powerful way to connect with others, reduce stigma, and advocate for change.

In conclusion, personal stories and experiences play a valuable role in increasing understanding and reducing stigma around ADHD. They can provide a sense of community and support for individuals living with the condition, and can also be a powerful tool in raising awareness and advocating for policy change. While personal stories are not a substitute for scientific research and evidence-based treatment, they can provide important context and nuance to our understanding of ADHD.

Insights from individuals living with ADHD

Attention-deficit/hyperactivity disorder (ADHD) can present unique challenges for individuals who have it, affecting many areas of their lives, including education, work, and relationships. However, those who have ADHD can also provide valuable insights into their experiences and offer tips and strategies for managing the condition. Here, we will explore some of these insights and provide a glimpse into the lives of individuals living with ADHD.

Firstly, it is important to recognize that ADHD is not a one-size-fits-all condition. Each person who has ADHD may experience it differently, with varying symptoms and levels of severity. Some may struggle primarily with hyperactivity and impulsivity, while others may struggle with inattention and difficulty with organization and time management. Additionally, co-occurring conditions such as anxiety and depression can exacerbate the challenges of living with ADHD.

Despite these challenges, individuals with ADHD often demonstrate creativity, energy, and a unique way of looking at the world. Many describe a strong sense of curiosity and a tendency to hyperfocus on topics that interest them, often leading to a depth of knowledge and expertise in specific areas. However, this hyperfocus can also make it difficult to shift attention to less interesting tasks, leading to procrastination and difficulty with completing tasks.

One strategy that many individuals with ADHD find helpful is breaking tasks down into smaller, more manageable steps. This can help to reduce the overwhelm and anxiety that can come with facing a large, complex task. Others find that creating structure and routine can help to provide a sense of control and reduce the likelihood of forgetfulness or disorganization.

In terms of medication, some individuals with ADHD report finding significant relief from symptoms with the use of stimulant medications such as Adderall or Ritalin. However, others may find the side effects intolerable or prefer to manage their symptoms with non-pharmacological approaches such as therapy or lifestyle changes.

It is important to note that the experience of living with ADHD can also be impacted by factors such as gender, race, and socioeconomic status. For example, women with ADHD may be more likely to go undiagnosed or misdiagnosed, as their symptoms may present differently than those traditionally associated with ADHD. Additionally, individuals from lower socioeconomic backgrounds may face additional barriers to accessing resources and support for managing their symptoms.

Despite these challenges, there is a growing community of individuals with ADHD who are sharing their stories, advocating for greater awareness and understanding of the condition, and providing support for others who are navigating their own experiences. Online communities, such as social media groups and forums, can be particularly helpful for connecting with others who understand the unique challenges of living with ADHD.

In conclusion, living with ADHD can present unique challenges, but it is important to remember that each individual's experience is unique. Strategies for managing symptoms can vary widely and may involve a combination of medication, therapy, lifestyle changes, and support from friends and family. By sharing their stories and insights, individuals with

ADHD can help to reduce stigma and provide a valuable perspective on living with this condition.

Overcoming challenges and celebrating successes

Overcoming challenges and celebrating successes are two important aspects of living with ADHD. ADHD can present various challenges in different areas of life, including education, work, and relationships. However, it is important to remember that there are ways to overcome these challenges and celebrate successes, no matter how small they may seem.

One common challenge for individuals with ADHD is managing time and staying organized. This can be especially challenging in academic settings, where students with ADHD may struggle to keep up with assignments, deadlines, and studying. One strategy for overcoming this challenge is to use a planner or a scheduling app to keep track of assignments and due dates. Breaking down larger assignments into smaller tasks and setting realistic goals can also help individuals with ADHD manage their time more effectively.

Another challenge for individuals with ADHD is staying focused and avoiding distractions. This can be particularly difficult in work settings, where distractions such as emails, phone calls, and meetings can interfere with productivity. One strategy for overcoming this challenge is to create a distraction-free work environment. This can involve minimizing interruptions, using noise-cancelling headphones, and setting aside specific times for checking emails and taking breaks.

In relationships, individuals with ADHD may struggle with communication and maintaining focus during conversations. They may also be more impulsive or forgetful, which can lead to misunderstandings or missed appointments. One strategy for overcoming these challenges is to practice active listening and mindfulness. This can involve being fully present during conversations, repeating important information to ensure understanding, and taking a moment to think before responding to avoid impulsive reactions.

Despite these challenges, individuals with ADHD can still achieve success in various areas of life. Celebrating successes, no matter how small they may seem, is important for maintaining motivation and building self-esteem. This can involve setting achievable goals, such as completing a project or assignment, and acknowledging progress along the way.

It is also important for individuals with ADHD to recognize their strengths and unique abilities. ADHD can present challenges, but it can also come with strengths such as creativity, adaptability, and problem-solving skills. Recognizing and building on these strengths can help individuals with ADHD achieve success and feel more confident in their abilities.

Additionally, seeking support from others can be helpful in overcoming challenges and achieving success. This can involve reaching out to friends, family members, or support groups for encouragement and guidance. Therapy and counseling can also be beneficial in providing strategies for managing symptoms and addressing any emotional or psychological difficulties related to ADHD.

In conclusion, overcoming challenges and celebrating successes are important aspects of living with ADHD. While individuals with ADHD may face various challenges in different areas of life, there are strategies and supports available to help them manage symptoms and achieve success. By recognizing their strengths, setting achievable goals, and seeking support from others, individuals with ADHD can navigate the challenges of daily life and celebrate their successes, no matter how small they may seem.

Inspiring stories of resilience and achievement

ADHD is a condition that can present unique challenges in daily life, such as difficulty with organization, time management, and focus. However, many individuals with ADHD have found ways to overcome these challenges and achieve success in various areas of their lives. These inspiring stories of resilience and achievement can serve as examples of hope and motivation for others with ADHD.

One such example is Michael Phelps, the most decorated Olympian of all time with 28 medals, including 23 gold. Phelps has spoken openly about his struggles with ADHD and how swimming provided an outlet for his hyperactivity and helped him focus his energy in a positive way. He has credited his success to his ability to set goals, create structure in his training and competition schedules, and use visualization techniques to improve his performance.

Another example is Simone Biles, a gymnastics superstar and multiple Olympic gold medalist. Biles was diagnosed with ADHD at a young age and has spoken about how her diagnosis has impacted her life and career. She has credited her success to her strong work ethic, determination, and ability to focus on the task at hand. Biles has also used her platform to advocate for mental health and destigmatize conditions like ADHD.

Entrepreneur and founder of Virgin Group, Richard Branson, has also spoken openly about his struggles with ADHD and dyslexia. Despite facing challenges in school and struggling with traditional learning methods, Branson found success by leveraging his strengths, such as creativity and a willingness to take risks. He has credited his success to his ability to delegate tasks, surround himself with supportive people, and maintain a positive attitude.

These examples show that individuals with ADHD can achieve great success in a variety of fields. However, it is important to note that each person's journey is unique and there is no one-size-fits-all approach to managing ADHD symptoms. It is also important to recognize that for some individuals, ADHD can present significant challenges that require professional support and treatment.

In addition to high-profile individuals, there are also many inspiring stories of everyday people with ADHD who have overcome challenges and achieved success in their own way. For example, a college student with ADHD may struggle with time management and organization, but find success by breaking tasks into smaller, manageable pieces and using technology to set reminders and stay on track. A small business owner with ADHD may struggle with multitasking, but find success by delegating tasks and focusing on the most important priorities.

It is important for individuals with ADHD to celebrate their successes, no matter how small, and to seek support and guidance when facing challenges. Support can come from a variety of sources, including family, friends, mental health professionals, and support groups. By connecting with others who understand the challenges of ADHD, individuals can find a sense of community and reduce feelings of isolation.

In conclusion, ADHD can present unique challenges in daily life, but with the right support and tools, individuals with ADHD can overcome these challenges and achieve success in various areas of their lives. The stories of high-profile individuals like Michael Phelps, Simone Biles, and Richard Branson can serve as inspiration for others with ADHD, while everyday people with ADHD can find success in their own unique ways. It is important for individuals with ADHD to celebrate their successes, seek support when facing challenges, and connect with others who understand their experiences.

Chapter Twenty-Two

ADHD and Creativity

ADHD, or Attention Deficit Hyperactivity Disorder, is a neurodevelopmental disorder that affects many aspects of an individual's life. It can cause difficulties with attention, impulsivity, and hyperactivity, and can impact both academic and social functioning. However, ADHD is not all negative, and some studies suggest that it may have some positive effects on creativity.

Creativity is defined as the ability to generate novel and useful ideas or solutions. It is an important aspect of many professions, including art, music, writing, and science. While there is no clear consensus on the relationship between ADHD and creativity, many individuals with ADHD report being highly creative.

One theory suggests that ADHD may increase creativity by allowing individuals to think outside the box and take risks. Individuals with ADHD often struggle with traditional academic tasks, such as memorization and rote learning. However, this difficulty can also lead them to explore alternative ways of learning and thinking, which can result in novel and innovative ideas.

Research has found a correlation between ADHD and creativity in some domains. For example, one study found that individuals with ADHD scored higher on a measure of creative achievement than non-ADHD controls. Another study found that children with ADHD generated more creative solutions on a divergent thinking task than non-ADHD controls.

It is important to note that while ADHD may be associated with creativity, not all individuals with ADHD are creative, and not all creative individuals have ADHD. Furthermore, creativity is a complex construct that can be influenced by a variety of factors, including environmental and genetic factors.

Despite the potential benefits of ADHD on creativity, individuals with ADHD still face many challenges in their daily lives. These challenges can include difficulty with organization and time management, social relationships, and academic and professional success. Therefore, it is important to focus on strategies to manage ADHD symptoms and improve overall functioning.

One important strategy for managing ADHD symptoms is medication. Stimulant medications such as Ritalin and Adderall have been shown to improve attention and reduce hyperactivity and impulsivity in individuals with ADHD. These medications can also improve academic and professional success and may indirectly contribute to creativity by reducing distractions and allowing for sustained focus.

In addition to medication, there are several other strategies that can help individuals with ADHD manage their symptoms and improve functioning. These strategies include cognitive-behavioral therapy, organizational skills training, and social skills training. Cognitive-behavioral therapy can help individuals with ADHD manage negative thoughts and behaviors, while organizational skills training can improve time management and reduce clutter and distractions. Social skills training can help individuals with ADHD improve communication and relationship skills.

In conclusion, ADHD and creativity are complex constructs that can be influenced by a variety of factors. While some studies suggest that ADHD may increase creativity, it is important to focus on managing ADHD symptoms and improving overall functioning. Strategies such as medication, therapy, and skills training can be effective in managing ADHD symptoms and improving quality of life for individuals with ADHD.

The connection between ADHD and creative thinking

ADHD, or Attention-Deficit/Hyperactivity Disorder, is a neurodevelopmental disorder that is characterized by symptoms such as impulsivity, inattention, and hyperactivity. Although these symptoms can pose significant challenges in daily life, many individuals with ADHD have also been noted to have exceptional creative abilities. This connection between ADHD and creativity has been a topic of interest among researchers and has led to a growing understanding of how the disorder can impact creativity.

One of the main theories behind the relationship between ADHD and creativity is the idea of divergent thinking. Divergent thinking is a cognitive process that involves generating a wide variety of ideas in response to a given stimulus. This type of thinking is thought to be a key component of creativity, as it allows individuals to come up with unique solutions and approaches to problems. Individuals with ADHD have been found to excel in tasks that require divergent thinking, such as brainstorming, idea generation, and creative writing.

Another factor that contributes to the link between ADHD and creativity is the hyperactive nature of the disorder. Individuals with ADHD often have high levels of energy and can become easily bored. This can lead to a need for constant stimulation and new experiences, which can fuel creativity. In addition, the impulsivity that is often associated with ADHD can lead individuals to take risks and explore new ideas that others may not have considered.

However, while ADHD can have a positive impact on creativity, it can also present unique challenges. For example, individuals with ADHD may struggle with organization and time management, which can make it difficult to pursue creative endeavors. In addition, the impulsivity and distractibility associated with the disorder can make it hard to stay focused on a project, leading to unfinished or incomplete work.

Despite these challenges, many individuals with ADHD have found ways to use their creativity to their advantage. Some have channeled their energy and ideas into successful careers in fields such as art, music, and writing. Others have found that creative hobbies such as painting, crafting, or playing music can provide an outlet for their restless energy and help them cope with the challenges of the disorder.

While the link between ADHD and creativity is still being explored, it is clear that the disorder can have a significant impact on an individual's ability to think creatively. By understanding this connection and finding ways to manage the challenges that come with ADHD, individuals with the disorder can harness their creative potential and find success in their personal and professional lives.

Strategies for channeling ADHD-related strengths

ADHD is often associated with difficulties such as impulsivity, distractibility, and hyperactivity. However, it is also associated with a number of strengths that are often overlooked. People with ADHD tend to be creative, spontaneous, and innovative. They are often excellent problem solvers and can think outside the box. However, it can be challenging for people with ADHD to channel their strengths and use them to their advantage. Below we will we will explore some strategies for doing just that.

The first step in channeling ADHD-related strengths is to recognize and embrace them. Many people with ADHD grow up feeling like their differences make them inadequate, and as a result, they may not recognize their strengths. By identifying and embracing their strengths, people with ADHD can develop a more positive self-image and gain the confidence to tackle challenges.

One of the most significant strengths associated with ADHD is creativity. People with ADHD often have a unique perspective on the world and can think in unconventional ways. This creativity can be harnessed in various ways, from artistic pursuits to problem-solving in the workplace. It's essential to recognize that creativity doesn't have to be limited to traditional artistic pursuits. People with ADHD can apply their creativity to many areas of their lives, from cooking to home décor to entrepreneurship.

Another strength that people with ADHD often possess is an ability to hyperfocus. Hyperfocus is an intense level of concentration that can occur when someone with ADHD becomes engrossed in a task they enjoy or find stimulating. When harnessed correctly, this hyperfocus can be a valuable tool. For example, someone with ADHD may be able to work on a project for an extended period without becoming distracted, allowing them to complete the task more quickly than someone without ADHD.

To channel their strengths, people with ADHD must learn to manage their weaknesses. This includes strategies such as breaking tasks into smaller, more manageable pieces, utilizing organizational tools such as calendars and to-do lists, and learning to recognize and avoid distractions. By managing their weaknesses, people with ADHD can free up more mental space to focus on their strengths.

Another crucial aspect of channeling strengths is finding the right environment. People with ADHD often struggle in environments that are too rigid or too chaotic. It's important to find a balance that allows them to work in an environment that is both structured enough to keep them on track but flexible enough to allow them to be creative.

Finally, people with ADHD must learn to advocate for themselves. This means communicating with others about their strengths and weaknesses and asking for accommodations when necessary. For example, someone with ADHD may need to request extra time to complete a task or a quieter workspace to minimize distractions.

In conclusion, people with ADHD often possess unique strengths that can be channeled in positive ways. To do so, it's essential to recognize and embrace these strengths, manage weaknesses, find the right environment, and advocate for oneself. By doing so, people with ADHD can harness their creativity, problem-solving skills, and hyperfocus to achieve success in all areas of their lives.

Success stories of creative individuals with ADHD

ADHD is often seen as a disadvantage or a hindrance to success, but for many individuals with ADHD, it can actually be a catalyst for creativity and innovation. The connection between ADHD and creativity has been noted for decades, and there are many examples of successful people with ADHD who have harnessed their unique cognitive abilities to achieve great things.

One of the key characteristics of ADHD is a tendency toward impulsivity and distractibility. While these traits can be challenging in certain situations, they can also contribute to divergent thinking and the ability to generate new and innovative ideas. Individuals with ADHD are often able to think outside the box and see connections between seemingly unrelated concepts. This can be particularly valuable in creative fields such as art, music, writing, and design.

Research has shown that people with ADHD may be particularly skilled at tasks that involve divergent thinking, which is the ability to come up with multiple possible solutions to a problem. One study found that adults with ADHD outperformed neurotypical adults on a test of creative problem-solving, suggesting that their impulsivity and ability to generate multiple ideas quickly may give them an advantage in certain situations.

Of course, creativity alone is not enough to achieve success. Individuals with ADHD may struggle with executive function skills such as planning, organization, and time management, which can make it difficult to bring creative ideas to fruition. However, with the right support and strategies, it is possible to channel ADHD-related strengths into productive and successful endeavors.

One of the most important strategies for leveraging ADHD-related strengths is to focus on areas of interest and passion. Many people with ADHD are able to hyperfocus on tasks that they find engaging or enjoyable, and this can be a valuable asset when it comes to pursuing creative projects. By tapping into their natural enthusiasm and curiosity, individuals with ADHD can often find new and innovative ways to approach creative challenges.

Another key strategy is to develop effective time management and organizational skills. This can be particularly important for creative individuals, who may struggle with self-discipline and procrastination. By setting clear goals, breaking tasks into manageable chunks, and using tools such as calendars and to-do lists, people with ADHD can stay on track and ensure that their creative work is completed on time and to a high standard.

It is also important to recognize and manage the potential downsides of ADHD, such as impulsivity and distractibility. While these traits can be assets in certain situations, they can also be liabilities if not managed effectively. People with ADHD may need to develop specific strategies to stay focused and avoid distractions, such as working in a quiet environment or using noise-cancelling headphones. Additionally, it may be helpful to work with a coach or therapist who specializes in ADHD to develop personalized strategies for managing symptoms and maximizing strengths.

There are many examples of successful people with ADHD who have harnessed their creativity and channeled their energy into productive endeavors. Some famous examples include musician Justin Timberlake, author and motivational speaker Dr. Ned Hallowell, and entrepreneur Sir Richard Branson. These individuals have all found ways to leverage their ADHD-related strengths to achieve success and make a positive impact in their respective fields.

In addition to these high-profile examples, there are countless people with ADHD who are using their creativity to achieve success in less publicized fields. From artists and writers to entrepreneurs and innovators, there are many individuals with ADHD who are thriving in their chosen fields by tapping into their natural creativity and energy.

Chapter Twenty-Three

Embracing Neurodiversity

1 . Embracing Neurodiversity: Understanding and Celebrating Differences

Neurodiversity is a term used to describe the wide variation in neurological differences that occur among individuals. It is based on the belief that these differences should be recognized, valued and respected, and that there is no "normal" or "abnormal" way to be neurologically diverse. Neurodiversity is not limited to ADHD, but it is an important aspect of ADHD acceptance and understanding. Below we will explore the concept of neurodiversity, how it relates to ADHD, and why embracing neurodiversity is important.

Neurodiversity encompasses a wide range of neurological differences, including autism, ADHD, dyslexia, and Tourette's syndrome, among others. These differences can be seen as a form of diversity, similar to cultural, linguistic, or gender diversity. Neurodiversity is not a disorder or a medical condition; it is a natural variation of the human experience. Neurodivergent individuals have unique strengths and challenges that should be recognized and celebrated.

ADHD is one of the most common neurodivergent conditions, affecting around 6-9% of children and 2-5% of adults worldwide. It is characterized by inattention, hyperactivity, and impulsivity. However, ADHD is not just a disorder of attention and behavior; it is a complex neurological condition that affects the way individuals process information, emotions, and relationships.

For many years, ADHD was seen as a purely negative condition, and individuals with ADHD were often labeled as lazy, disorganized, or difficult. However, recent research has shown that ADHD is not just a disability; it can also be a source of creativity, innovation, and success. Neurodivergent individuals have unique strengths that can be harnessed to create positive change in the world.

One of the key principles of neurodiversity is the acceptance of differences. Neurodivergent individuals have a right to be different and to be accepted for who they are. This means recognizing that there is no one "normal" way to be, and that diversity should be celebrated rather than stigmatized. Acceptance means understanding that neurodivergent individuals have different needs, preferences, and abilities, and that these differences should be accommodated and respected.

Embracing neurodiversity also means recognizing that neurodivergent individuals have unique strengths that can be leveraged to create positive change. For example, many individuals with ADHD are highly creative and innovative, and have a natural ability to think outside the box. They are often able to come up with novel solutions to complex problems, and have a unique perspective on the world. These strengths should be recognized and celebrated, and individuals with ADHD should be given opportunities to use their strengths in meaningful ways.

Another important aspect of neurodiversity is the concept of inclusion. This means creating an environment where all individuals, regardless of their neurological differences, are able to participate fully and contribute their unique perspectives and abilities. Inclusion means recognizing that everyone has something to offer, and that everyone should be given the opportunity to succeed.

Finally, embracing neurodiversity means challenging the negative stereotypes and misconceptions that surround neurodivergent individuals. This means recognizing that ADHD is not just a disorder of attention and behavior, but a complex neurological condition that affects every aspect of an individual's life. It means recognizing that neurodivergent individuals are not broken or defective, but unique and valuable members of society.

In conclusion, embracing neurodiversity is an important step towards creating a more inclusive and accepting society. It means recognizing and celebrating the unique strengths and abilities of neurodivergent individuals, and challenging the negative stereotypes and misconceptions that surround them.

The concept of neurodiversity and its importance in understanding ADHD

The concept of neurodiversity has gained popularity in recent years, especially within the ADHD community. It suggests that differences in brain function and development should be celebrated, rather than pathologized. Neurodiversity is based on the idea that everyone's brain works differently and that these differences are essential to the diversity of human experience.

Neurodiversity is particularly relevant to ADHD, a condition that affects millions of people around the world. ADHD is a developmental disorder that impacts the way the brain processes information, particularly in areas related to attention, focus, and impulse control. Those with ADHD may struggle with tasks that require sustained attention, planning, and organization, and can often be easily distracted.

Traditionally, ADHD has been viewed as a disorder that needs to be fixed or cured. This perspective has led to a medical model of treatment, primarily based on medication and behavioral interventions. However, the neurodiversity approach challenges this notion and emphasizes the need to embrace the strengths and unique qualities of individuals with ADHD.

The concept of neurodiversity highlights that ADHD is not a deficit in attention, but rather a difference in the way attention is paid. Individuals with ADHD may excel in areas that require divergent thinking, such as problem-solving, creativity, and innovation. This unique cognitive profile can be an asset in fields such as art, science, and entrepreneurship, where a different perspective can lead to breakthroughs and success.

Furthermore, the neurodiversity approach encourages us to move beyond the medical model of ADHD treatment and support. Instead of treating ADHD as a disorder, neurodiversity advocates for creating an environment that values and supports individuals with ADHD. This includes reducing stigma, promoting inclusion and diversity, and providing accommodations and support for individuals with ADHD in education and the workplace.

Embracing neurodiversity is essential for promoting mental health and well-being among individuals with ADHD. Acceptance and understanding of neurodiversity can lead to improved self-esteem, reduced anxiety, and better mental health outcomes. When individuals with ADHD are encouraged to embrace their differences and strengths, they are more likely to feel empowered and confident in their abilities.

It is important to note that embracing neurodiversity does not mean ignoring or downplaying the challenges that individuals with ADHD face. It simply means acknowledging that ADHD is not a deficit, but a difference. By recognizing and valuing these differences, we can create a more inclusive and accepting society that celebrates diversity and promotes individual strengths.

In conclusion, the concept of neurodiversity is an essential framework for understanding ADHD. Rather than viewing ADHD as a disorder that needs to be cured, the neurodiversity approach emphasizes the unique cognitive profile and strengths of individuals with ADHD. Embracing neurodiversity can lead to improved mental health outcomes, reduced stigma, and a more inclusive and accepting society. It is time to move beyond the medical model of treatment and support for ADHD and to embrace the power of neurodiversity.

Challenging stigma and embracing different ways of thinking

Attention Deficit Hyperactivity Disorder (ADHD) is a condition that affects approximately 10% of the population, and it is often associated with negative stereotypes such as being lazy, unmotivated, or unproductive. However, these stereotypes are far from the truth, and they only serve to perpetuate a harmful stigma surrounding ADHD. Instead of focusing on the negatives, it is important to embrace the concept of neurodiversity and challenge the stigma surrounding different ways of thinking.

Neurodiversity refers to the idea that neurological differences such as ADHD, autism, and dyslexia are not disorders but instead are natural variations in the human population. This concept is important because it challenges the traditional view of neurodivergent individuals as being abnormal or defective. Instead, it recognizes that every person has a unique brain and different ways of processing information.

When it comes to ADHD, the concept of neurodiversity is particularly important because it challenges the idea that ADHD is a purely negative condition. While ADHD can certainly present challenges, it also comes with many strengths and unique ways of thinking that can be incredibly valuable. For example, individuals with ADHD may be highly creative, energetic, and able to think outside the box. These are all traits that can be incredibly beneficial in certain situations, such as problem-solving or creative fields.

Challenging the stigma surrounding ADHD and embracing neurodiversity requires a shift in mindset. Instead of viewing ADHD as a negative condition, it is important to recognize that it is simply a different way of thinking. This means challenging negative stereotypes and assumptions about individuals with ADHD and recognizing the unique strengths that they bring to the table.

One way to challenge the stigma surrounding ADHD is to educate others about the condition. Many people may not be familiar with what ADHD is or how it affects individuals, and may instead rely on stereotypes and assumptions. By sharing information about ADHD and challenging these assumptions, it is possible to create a more understanding and accepting environment.

Another way to embrace neurodiversity is to focus on strengths rather than weaknesses. For example, instead of focusing on what an individual with ADHD struggles with, it is important to recognize their strengths and unique ways of thinking. By focusing on what they can do well and finding ways to channel their strengths, it is possible to create an environment that is more accommodating and supportive.

It is also important to create a more inclusive environment for individuals with ADHD. This means recognizing that certain traditional structures such as the 9-5 workday may not work well for everyone. Instead, it is important to be flexible and open to different ways of working and thinking. This could mean allowing individuals to work remotely or to have flexible hours, or simply being open to different ways of approaching tasks.

In addition to challenging stigma and embracing neurodiversity, it is also important to support and advocate for individuals with ADHD. This could mean advocating for more accommodations in the workplace or in educational settings, or simply being a supportive friend or family member. By creating a more supportive environment, individuals with ADHD can thrive and reach their full potential.

In conclusion, the concept of neurodiversity is an important one when it comes to ADHD. By recognizing that different ways of thinking are not disorders but instead natural variations in the human population, it is possible to challenge the stigma surrounding ADHD and embrace different ways of thinking. This requires a shift in mindset and a focus on strengths rather than weaknesses, as well as creating a more inclusive and supportive environment for individuals with ADHD. Ultimately, by embracing neurodiversity, we can create a world that is more understanding, accepting, and accommodating for everyone.

Advocating for a more inclusive and supportive society

ADHD, or attention-deficit/hyperactivity disorder, affects millions of individuals worldwide. It is a neurodevelopmental disorder that can affect people of all ages and can impact multiple areas of their lives, including social, academic, and occupational functioning. Despite being a well-known condition, individuals with ADHD still face a lot of stigma and discrimination in various aspects of their lives. Therefore, it is crucial to advocate for a more inclusive and supportive society that recognizes and accommodates the diverse needs of individuals with ADHD.

One of the primary ways to advocate for a more inclusive society is to educate people about ADHD. Many individuals still have a limited understanding of the condition, and they often rely on stereotypes and misinformation to form their opinions. Therefore, it is important to provide accurate information about ADHD, its symptoms, and its impact on individuals' lives. Educating people about the condition can help reduce stigma and encourage a more compassionate and understanding approach towards individuals with ADHD.

Another way to advocate for a more inclusive society is to promote awareness of the challenges individuals with ADHD face. These challenges can vary widely, depending on factors such as age, gender, and cultural background. Some common challenges that individuals with ADHD may face include difficulties with organization, time management, and impulse control. They may also experience difficulties with social interaction, such as making and maintaining friendships, due to their hyperactivity or inattention. Raising awareness of these challenges can help individuals with ADHD feel more understood and supported by their communities.

In addition to raising awareness of the challenges that individuals with ADHD face, it is also important to advocate for accommodations and support services that can help them succeed. For example, students with ADHD may benefit from extra time on exams or the use of assistive technology, such as speech-to-text software. Workplace accommodations, such as flexible work hours or the use of noise-canceling headphones, can also be beneficial for adults with ADHD. By advocating for these accommodations and support services, individuals with ADHD can have an equal opportunity to succeed and contribute to their communities.

Moreover, it is important to promote research and understanding of ADHD to develop better ways to support individuals with the condition. Research on ADHD is ongoing, and it is essential to keep up-to-date with the latest developments. By promoting research and understanding of ADHD, we can learn more about the condition's underlying causes and develop more effective treatment and support strategies.

Lastly, individuals with ADHD should be empowered to speak out and advocate for themselves. Encouraging individuals with ADHD to share their stories and experiences can help break down stereotypes and promote understanding of the condition. When individuals with ADHD speak out, they can also help advocate for changes in policies and attitudes that affect their lives. It is essential to create safe and supportive spaces where individuals with ADHD can share their experiences without fear of judgment or discrimination.

In conclusion, advocating for a more inclusive and supportive society for individuals with ADHD is crucial. It involves educating people about the condition, promoting awareness of the challenges individuals with ADHD face, advocating for accommodations and support services, promoting research and understanding of ADHD, and empowering individuals with ADHD to speak out and advocate for themselves. By working together to create a more inclusive and supportive society, we can help individuals with ADHD succeed and thrive in all aspects of their lives.

Chapter Twenty-Four

Mindfulness and ADHD

Mindfulness is a popular technique used to manage stress and anxiety, but it can also be an effective tool for individuals with ADHD. Mindfulness is the practice of focusing one's attention on the present moment and accepting it without judgment. It involves paying attention to thoughts and sensations as they arise, without getting caught up in them or reacting to them.

For individuals with ADHD, mindfulness can help improve focus and attention, reduce impulsivity and hyperactivity, and increase self-awareness. It can also help to reduce stress and anxiety, which are common co-occurring conditions in individuals with ADHD.

One of the main benefits of mindfulness for individuals with ADHD is that it helps to increase self-awareness. By paying attention to thoughts and sensations as they arise, individuals with ADHD can become more aware of their triggers and patterns of behavior. This can help them to identify when they are becoming distracted or overwhelmed, and take steps to refocus their attention.

Another benefit of mindfulness is that it can help to improve focus and attention. By practicing mindfulness regularly, individuals with ADHD can improve their ability to stay focused on tasks and ignore distractions. This can help to improve academic and work performance, as well as overall quality of life.

Mindfulness can also help to reduce impulsivity and hyperactivity, which are hallmark symptoms of ADHD. By learning to focus on the present moment and accept thoughts and sensations without judgment, individuals with ADHD can reduce impulsive and reactive behaviors.

In addition to these benefits, mindfulness can also help to reduce stress and anxiety, which are common co-occurring conditions in individuals with ADHD. By learning to focus on the present moment and accept thoughts and sensations without judgment, individuals with ADHD can reduce their levels of stress and anxiety, which can in turn improve their overall well-being.

There are many different ways to practice mindfulness, and individuals with ADHD may need to experiment with different techniques to find what works best for them. Some common mindfulness techniques include:

1. Breathing exercises: Focusing on the breath is a simple and effective way to practice mindfulness. By focusing on the sensations of the breath as it enters and leaves the body, individuals with ADHD can become more aware of their thoughts and sensations.

2. Body scan: A body scan involves focusing on each part of the body in turn, from the top of the head to the tips of the toes. This can help to increase self-awareness and reduce stress and tension in the body.

3. Mindful movement: Activities like yoga, tai chi, and walking can all be practiced mindfully, by focusing on the sensations of the body as it moves.

4. Mindful eating: Eating mindfully involves paying attention to the taste, texture, and sensations of food as it is consumed. This can help individuals with ADHD to slow down and become more aware of their eating habits.

In conclusion, mindfulness can be a valuable tool for individuals with ADHD. By improving focus and attention, reducing impulsivity and hyperactivity, and increasing self-awareness, mindfulness can help individuals with ADHD to manage their symptoms and improve their overall well-being. There are many different ways to practice mindfulness, and individuals with ADHD may need to experiment with different techniques to find what works best for them.

The benefits of mindfulness practices for individuals with ADHD

The practice of mindfulness has been gaining popularity as a means of improving mental health and overall wellbeing. Mindfulness involves being present in the moment, observing thoughts and feelings without judgment, and focusing on the present. For individuals with ADHD, who often struggle with impulsivity, distractibility, and emotional dysregulation, mindfulness can offer a number of benefits. Below we will we will explore the benefits of mindfulness practices for individuals with ADHD.

One of the main benefits of mindfulness for individuals with ADHD is the development of greater self-awareness. Through mindfulness practices, individuals with ADHD can learn to identify the thoughts and emotions that are contributing to their difficulties with attention and focus. They can also learn to recognize when they are becoming distracted or overwhelmed, and take steps to re-focus and re-engage with their tasks.

Mindfulness practices can also help individuals with ADHD develop greater emotional regulation. Individuals with ADHD may experience intense emotions that are difficult to manage, leading to impulsivity and mood swings. Mindfulness can help individuals with ADHD to develop a greater sense of emotional awareness and control, allowing them to respond to situations more effectively and reduce impulsive behaviors.

In addition, mindfulness practices can improve attention and focus, which are areas of difficulty for individuals with ADHD. By practicing mindfulness, individuals with ADHD can improve their ability to sustain attention, resist distractions, and switch between tasks more effectively. This can help them to be more productive and achieve their goals more effectively.

Another benefit of mindfulness for individuals with ADHD is stress reduction. Stress is a common trigger for ADHD symptoms, and individuals with ADHD may find it difficult to manage stress effectively. Mindfulness practices can help individuals with ADHD to develop greater resilience to stress, by teaching them to observe their thoughts and emotions without becoming overwhelmed by them. This can lead to greater calm and relaxation, reducing the likelihood of ADHD symptoms being triggered by stress.

Finally, mindfulness can improve overall wellbeing for individuals with ADHD. By promoting greater self-awareness, emotional regulation, attention, and stress reduction, mindfulness can help individuals with ADHD to feel more grounded, present, and fulfilled in their daily lives.

There are a number of mindfulness practices that can be beneficial for individuals with ADHD. Mindful breathing exercises involve focusing on the breath and observing thoughts and feelings as they arise. Body scan meditations involve systematically focusing on different parts of the body, observing sensations without judgment. Mindful movement practices such as yoga or tai chi can also be beneficial for individuals with ADHD, as they combine physical movement with mindfulness techniques.

It is important to note that mindfulness practices are not a substitute for medication or other treatments for ADHD. However, mindfulness can be a useful complement to other treatments, helping individuals with ADHD to develop greater self-awareness, emotional regulation, and attention skills. It is important for individuals with ADHD to work with a qualified healthcare provider to develop a comprehensive treatment plan that includes a range of interventions tailored to their individual needs.

In conclusion, mindfulness practices can offer a number of benefits for individuals with ADHD, including greater self-awareness, emotional regulation, attention, stress reduction, and overall wellbeing. By incorporating mindfulness into their daily lives, individuals with ADHD can develop greater resilience to the challenges of living with ADHD, and achieve greater fulfillment and success in their personal and professional lives.

Incorporating mindfulness into daily routines

Mindfulness is a practice that involves being fully present and engaged in the present moment without judgment. It has been found to be a beneficial tool for individuals with ADHD, as it can help to improve focus, attention, and impulse control. Below we will we will discuss the benefits of incorporating mindfulness practices into daily routines for individuals with ADHD.

One of the main benefits of mindfulness for individuals with ADHD is that it helps to improve focus and attention. ADHD is characterized by distractibility and difficulty maintaining attention on a task. Mindfulness practices such as meditation and deep breathing can help to train the brain to stay focused on the present moment, which can improve attention and reduce distractibility.

Another benefit of mindfulness for individuals with ADHD is that it can help to improve impulse control. Many individuals with ADHD struggle with impulsivity, which can lead to impulsive behaviors such as interrupting others or acting without thinking. Mindfulness practices can help to increase self-awareness and self-control, which can reduce impulsive behaviors.

In addition to improving focus and impulse control, mindfulness practices can also help to reduce stress and anxiety. Many individuals with ADHD experience high levels of stress and anxiety due to the challenges of living with the disorder. Mindfulness practices such as meditation and deep breathing can help to reduce stress and anxiety by promoting relaxation and calmness.

Incorporating mindfulness into daily routines can be a helpful tool for individuals with ADHD. Here are some strategies for incorporating mindfulness into daily routines:

1. Start small: Begin with short mindfulness practices such as taking a few deep breaths or doing a quick body scan. Gradually increase the length of the practice over time.

2. Set a daily reminder: Use a calendar or reminder app to schedule time for mindfulness practice each day.

3. Practice mindfulness during routine activities: Incorporate mindfulness into daily routines such as brushing teeth or taking a shower.

4. Find a mindfulness buddy: Partner with a friend or family member to practice mindfulness together and hold each other accountable.

5. Experiment with different mindfulness practices: Try different types of mindfulness practices such as meditation, deep breathing, or yoga to find what works best.

In conclusion, mindfulness practices can be a valuable tool for individuals with ADHD. By improving focus, impulse control, and reducing stress and anxiety, mindfulness can help to improve overall well-being and quality of life. By incorporating mindfulness into daily routines, individuals with ADHD can experience the benefits of mindfulness in a practical and sustainable way.

Mindfulness techniques specifically designed for ADHD

Mindfulness techniques are becoming increasingly popular as a way to help individuals with ADHD manage their symptoms. Mindfulness is a practice that involves paying attention to the present moment with openness, curiosity, and without judgment. It can help individuals with ADHD develop greater awareness of their thoughts, emotions, and behaviors, which can be helpful in reducing impulsivity, improving attention, and increasing emotional regulation.

For individuals with ADHD, it can be challenging to stay focused on the present moment and avoid getting distracted by thoughts, emotions, and external stimuli. Mindfulness techniques can help them train their minds to focus on the present moment, and to avoid getting caught up in distractions. There are several mindfulness techniques that are specifically designed for individuals with ADHD.

One such technique is called "mindful breathing." This involves focusing on the sensations of breathing, such as the feeling of air moving in and out of the nostrils. This technique can help individuals with ADHD slow down and regulate their breathing, which can have a calming effect on the mind and body. It can also help them to refocus their attention when they get distracted.

Another technique that can be helpful for individuals with ADHD is "body scan." This involves bringing attention to different parts of the body, and noticing any sensations that are present. This technique can help individuals with ADHD become more aware of their physical sensations, which can help them to stay grounded in the present moment. It can also help them to become more aware of any tension or discomfort in their bodies, which they can then work to release.

A third mindfulness technique that can be helpful for individuals with ADHD is "mindful walking." This involves walking slowly and intentionally, and focusing on the sensations of walking, such as the feeling of the feet on the ground. This technique can be helpful for individuals with ADHD who struggle with hyperactivity or restlessness. It can help them to release pent-up energy, while also helping them to stay focused on the present moment.

In addition to these techniques, there are also several mindfulness-based programs that have been specifically designed for individuals with ADHD. One such program is Mindful Schools, which is a mindfulness-based program that is designed for children with ADHD. The program teaches children mindfulness techniques that they can use to regulate their emotions, improve attention, and reduce stress.

Another program that has been specifically designed for individuals with ADHD is Mindfulness-Based Cognitive Therapy (MBCT). This program combines mindfulness techniques with cognitive-behavioral therapy to help individuals with ADHD develop greater awareness of their thoughts and emotions, and to change unhelpful patterns of thinking and behavior.

Research has shown that mindfulness techniques can be helpful for individuals with ADHD. One study found that adults with ADHD who participated in an eight-week mindfulness program showed improvements in attention and reduced hyperactivity. Another study found that children with ADHD who participated in a mindfulness-based program showed improvements in attention, emotional regulation, and social skills.

Incorporating mindfulness into daily routines can be helpful for individuals with ADHD. Some simple ways to incorporate mindfulness into daily life include taking a few deep breaths before starting a task, taking short mindful breaks throughout the day, and practicing mindfulness while engaging in routine activities such as brushing teeth or washing dishes.

In conclusion, mindfulness techniques can be a helpful tool for individuals with ADHD to manage their symptoms. Mindfulness-based programs, such as Mindful Schools and MBCT, have been specifically designed to help individuals with ADHD develop greater awareness of their thoughts, emotions, and behaviors, and to improve attention and emotional regulation. Mindfulness techniques such as mindful breathing, body scan, and mindful walking can be helpful in reducing impulsivity, improving attention, and increasing emotional regulation. Incorporating mindfulness into daily routines can be a simple and effective way for individuals with ADHD to improve their overall well-being.

Chapter Twenty-Five

Organization and Time Management

Organization and time management can be challenging for individuals with Attention Deficit Hyperactivity Disorder (ADHD). The disorder is characterized by symptoms of inattention, hyperactivity, and impulsivity that can interfere with a person's ability to stay organized and manage their time effectively. However, with the right strategies and tools, individuals with ADHD can learn to manage these difficulties and improve their daily functioning.

One of the most common challenges for individuals with ADHD is maintaining organization. Many individuals with ADHD struggle with keeping track of their belongings, completing tasks on time, and keeping their living and work spaces tidy. This can lead to feelings of overwhelm, stress, and anxiety. However, there are several strategies that can help individuals with ADHD stay organized and on top of their responsibilities.

One effective strategy is to create a daily schedule or routine. This can help individuals with ADHD structure their day and prioritize tasks. It is important to break tasks down into smaller, manageable steps and to set realistic goals for each day. Utilizing visual aids such as calendars, checklists, and to-do lists can also be helpful for staying organized.

Another effective strategy is to create designated spaces for important items and information. For example, having a designated spot for keys, wallet, and phone can help prevent misplacing them. Having a designated space for important papers and documents can also help prevent losing them.

In addition to organization, time management can also be a challenge for individuals with ADHD. Many individuals with ADHD struggle with procrastination, time estimation, and prioritizing tasks. However, there are several strategies that can help individuals with ADHD improve their time management skills.

One effective strategy is to break tasks down into smaller, more manageable steps. This can make tasks feel less overwhelming and can increase motivation to complete them. Another strategy is to prioritize tasks based on importance and urgency. This can help individuals with ADHD focus on the most important tasks first and prevent feeling overwhelmed.

Using time-tracking tools, such as a timer or stopwatch, can also be helpful for individuals with ADHD. These tools can help increase awareness of how much time is spent on tasks and can help with time estimation and staying on track.

Technology can also be a useful tool for individuals with ADHD. There are many apps and software programs designed specifically for organization and time management, such as calendars, to-do lists, and reminder apps. These tools can help individuals with ADHD stay on top of their responsibilities and prevent forgetfulness.

Overall, improving organization and time management skills can greatly benefit individuals with ADHD. It can help reduce feelings of overwhelm and stress, increase productivity and motivation, and improve daily functioning. Utilizing strategies such as creating a routine, using visual aids, breaking tasks down, and using technology can all be helpful in improving organization and time management for individuals with ADHD.

Strategies for improving organization and time management skills

Attention Deficit Hyperactivity Disorder (ADHD) is a neurodevelopmental disorder that can significantly impact an individual's ability to organize their thoughts, tasks, and time effectively. This can lead to difficulties in achieving academic and professional success, completing daily tasks, and managing relationships. However, there are several strategies that individuals with ADHD can use to improve their organization and time management skills, allowing them to achieve their goals and maximize their potential.

One of the most effective strategies for improving organization and time management skills is to establish a routine. This involves setting aside specific times each day for completing tasks, such as studying, working, exercising, and socializing. By establishing a routine, individuals with ADHD can ensure that they are making progress toward their goals each day, while also avoiding the overwhelming feeling that can come with attempting to complete all tasks at once. It is important to note that while routines can be helpful, it is also essential to allow for some flexibility, as unexpected events can arise.

Another strategy for improving organization and time management skills is to break tasks down into smaller, more manageable steps. This can be accomplished by creating a to-do list, which can help individuals with ADHD prioritize their tasks and stay on track. It is essential to break down each task into smaller steps, allowing for a sense of accomplishment as each step is completed. By setting achievable goals and celebrating each small success, individuals with ADHD can improve their motivation and self-confidence, leading to greater overall success.

In addition to establishing a routine and breaking down tasks into smaller steps, there are several other strategies that individuals with ADHD can use to improve their organization and time management skills. One strategy is to eliminate distractions, such as turning off cell phones, closing unnecessary web browsers, and working in a quiet environment. This can help individuals with ADHD stay focused and on-task, allowing them to complete tasks more efficiently. Another strategy is to use tools such as calendars, timers, and alarms, which can help individuals with ADHD stay on schedule and avoid procrastination.

It is also important for individuals with ADHD to recognize their strengths and weaknesses when it comes to organization and time management. For example, some individuals with ADHD may have difficulty remembering deadlines, while others may struggle with keeping their workspace organized. By identifying these strengths and weaknesses, individuals with ADHD can develop strategies that are tailored to their unique needs, allowing them to maximize their strengths and overcome their weaknesses.

Finally, it is essential for individuals with ADHD to seek support when needed. This can involve seeking help from family members, friends, or coworkers, or seeking professional help from a therapist or coach. By working with others, individuals with ADHD can receive encouragement, accountability, and guidance, helping them stay on track and achieve their goals.

In conclusion, individuals with ADHD can improve their organization and time management skills by establishing a routine, breaking down tasks into smaller steps, eliminating distractions, using tools such as calendars and timers, recognizing their strengths and weaknesses, and seeking support when needed. By implementing these strategies, individuals with ADHD can overcome the challenges associated with the disorder and achieve their full potential.

Tools and techniques for managing ADHD-related challenges

Attention-deficit/hyperactivity disorder (ADHD) can pose significant challenges for individuals in their daily lives. Some of the most common challenges include difficulty with organization, time management, and focusing on tasks. Fortunately, there are a variety of tools and techniques that can help individuals with ADHD manage these challenges and improve their overall quality of life.

One of the most effective tools for managing ADHD-related challenges is a planner or organizational system. This can include a paper planner, a digital calendar, or a combination of both. The key is to find a system that works for the individual and to consistently use it to plan out tasks and activities. This can help with time management, as well as providing a visual reminder of upcoming tasks.

Breaking tasks down into smaller, more manageable steps can also be helpful for individuals with ADHD. This can make tasks feel less overwhelming and more achievable. Additionally, it can be helpful to prioritize tasks and focus on completing the most important or urgent ones first.

Another technique for managing ADHD-related challenges is to use visual aids, such as color coding or labeling. This can be particularly helpful for organizing items, such as files or school supplies, and can help individuals quickly and easily find what they need.

Technology can also be a useful tool for managing ADHD-related challenges. There are a variety of apps and software programs specifically designed for individuals with ADHD, such as reminder apps and focus timers. Additionally, digital organization tools, such as Trello or Evernote, can be helpful for managing tasks and projects.

Incorporating exercise and movement into daily routines can also be helpful for managing ADHD-related challenges. Exercise can help increase focus and attention, as well as reduce anxiety and stress. This can be particularly helpful for individuals with ADHD, who may struggle with staying focused or managing their emotions.

Mindfulness practices, such as meditation and deep breathing exercises, can also be helpful for managing ADHD-related challenges. Mindfulness can help increase self-awareness and focus, as well as reduce anxiety and stress. Additionally, mindfulness practices can be helpful for managing impulsivity and improving emotional regulation.

It is important to remember that managing ADHD-related challenges can be an ongoing process and may require some trial and error to find what works best for each individual. It can also be helpful to seek support from a mental health professional, such as a therapist or psychiatrist, who can provide guidance and support in managing ADHD-related challenges.

In conclusion, there are a variety of tools and techniques available to help individuals with ADHD manage challenges related to organization, time management, and focus. These include using planners or organizational systems, breaking tasks down into smaller steps, using visual aids, utilizing technology, incorporating exercise and movement, and practicing mindfulness. With persistence and support, individuals with ADHD can learn to effectively manage their symptoms and lead fulfilling lives.

Developing habits that promote long-term success

Attention Deficit Hyperactivity Disorder (ADHD) is a neurological condition that affects an individual's ability to sustain attention, control impulses, and manage hyperactivity or restlessness. ADHD can affect individuals of all ages, and it can have significant impacts on academic and professional success, relationships, and overall quality of life. While ADHD can present unique challenges, there are several strategies that individuals with ADHD can use to develop habits that promote long-term success.

One of the most effective ways for individuals with ADHD to promote long-term success is by establishing routines and habits. Establishing routines can be difficult for individuals with ADHD, but it can help to reduce the impact of symptoms such as procrastination and forgetfulness. Routines can help individuals with ADHD to create structure and predictability, which can help to reduce anxiety and overwhelm. Some examples of routines that can be helpful for individuals with ADHD include creating a consistent sleep schedule, setting aside time each day for exercise, and developing a routine for completing daily tasks.

In addition to establishing routines, individuals with ADHD can benefit from developing strategies for managing distractions. Distractions can be particularly challenging for individuals with ADHD, as they can easily become hyper-focused on activities that are not productive. One effective strategy for managing distractions is to limit exposure to potential distractions, such as social media or other forms of technology. It can also be helpful to create an environment that is conducive to focus, such as by removing clutter and creating a quiet workspace.

Another important strategy for individuals with ADHD is to break down large tasks into smaller, more manageable steps. ADHD can make it difficult to focus on long-term goals or projects, but breaking them down into smaller steps can make them more approachable. This can help to reduce the feeling of overwhelm and increase the likelihood of success. It can also be helpful to set deadlines for each step in the process, which can help to create a sense of urgency and promote accountability.

In addition to establishing routines and managing distractions, individuals with ADHD can benefit from developing strategies for improving memory and organization skills. ADHD can make it challenging to remember important details, such as deadlines or appointments, and to keep track of tasks and responsibilities. One effective strategy for improving memory and organization skills is to use visual aids, such as color-coded calendars or to-do lists. It can also be helpful to use technology, such as smartphone apps, to set reminders or to keep track of important information.

Finally, individuals with ADHD can benefit from seeking support and guidance from others. This can include seeking out professional support, such as working with a therapist or coach who specializes in ADHD, or seeking support from peers who have similar experiences. Support groups can be particularly helpful, as they provide a space for individuals with ADHD to connect with others who understand their challenges and experiences. It can also be helpful to involve family members or friends in the process, as they can provide encouragement and accountability.

In conclusion, ADHD can present unique challenges for individuals of all ages, but there are several strategies that can help individuals with ADHD to develop habits that promote long-term success. These strategies include establishing routines, managing distractions, breaking down large tasks into smaller steps, improving memory and organization skills, and seeking support and guidance from others. By implementing these strategies, individuals with ADHD can increase their likelihood of success in academic, professional, and personal pursuits.

Chapter Twenty-Six

ADHD and Emotional Regulation

ADHD, or Attention-Deficit/Hyperactivity Disorder, is a neurodevelopmental disorder that affects people's ability to focus, stay organized, and control their impulses. One of the lesser-known symptoms of ADHD is difficulty with emotional regulation. Emotional regulation refers to a person's ability to manage their emotions in response to different situations. This includes the ability to recognize and label emotions, to regulate the intensity and duration of emotional responses, and to use effective coping strategies when experiencing negative emotions. Below we will we will explore the relationship between ADHD and emotional regulation, as well as strategies for improving emotional regulation skills in people with ADHD.

The Link Between ADHD and Emotional Dysregulation

Emotional dysregulation is a common feature of ADHD. Studies have found that people with ADHD are more likely to experience intense and prolonged emotional responses, difficulty identifying emotions, and difficulty using effective coping strategies to manage negative emotions. This can result in problems with mood, relationships, and overall quality of life. Children with ADHD are more likely to experience emotional and behavioral problems, including irritability, anxiety, depression, and aggression. Adults with ADHD may struggle with emotional regulation in the workplace, in relationships, and in social situations.

One reason for the link between ADHD and emotional dysregulation is the role of the prefrontal cortex, a part of the brain that is responsible for executive functions such as attention, impulse control, and emotional regulation. People with ADHD have been found to have reduced prefrontal cortex activity compared to neurotypical individuals, which can affect their ability to regulate emotions. Additionally, the presence of comorbid conditions such as anxiety and depression can exacerbate emotional dysregulation in people with ADHD.

Strategies for Improving Emotional Regulation in ADHD

Fortunately, there are many strategies and techniques that can help people with ADHD improve their emotional regulation skills. Here are some strategies that may be helpful:

Mindfulness-Based Interventions

Mindfulness-based interventions, such as mindfulness meditation, have been shown to improve emotional regulation in people with ADHD. Mindfulness involves paying attention to the present moment without judgment, which can help people with ADHD become more aware of their emotions and better able to regulate them. Mindfulness can also improve attention and executive function, which can in turn improve emotional regulation.

Cognitive Behavioral Therapy

Cognitive-behavioral therapy (CBT) is a type of therapy that can help people with ADHD develop more effective coping strategies for managing emotions. CBT focuses on changing negative patterns of thought and behavior, and can help people with ADHD develop skills such as cognitive restructuring, problem-solving, and relaxation techniques. CBT has been shown to be effective in improving emotional regulation in both children and adults with ADHD.

Exercise and Physical Activity

Physical activity has been shown to improve emotional regulation in people with ADHD. Exercise can help reduce stress and anxiety, improve mood, and increase self-esteem. Exercise has also been shown to increase the production of endorphins, the body's natural feel-good chemicals.

Sleep Hygiene

Sleep is essential for emotional regulation, and people with ADHD often struggle with sleep difficulties. Improving sleep hygiene can be an effective strategy for improving emotional regulation in people with ADHD. This includes setting a consistent bedtime and wake time, creating a sleep-conducive environment, and avoiding screens before bedtime.

Medication

In some cases, medication may be necessary to improve emotional dysregulation in people with ADHD. Medications such as stimulants and non-stimulants can help improve attention and impulse control, which can in turn improve emotional regulation. However, medication is not a standalone treatment and should be used in conjunction with other strategies and interventions.

Understanding the connection between ADHD and emotional regulation

Attention-deficit/hyperactivity disorder (ADHD) is a neurodevelopmental disorder that affects approximately 5-10% of children and 2-5% of adults globally. One of the most common co-occurring symptoms of ADHD is difficulty with emotional regulation, which can lead to impulsivity, outbursts, and difficulty managing stress. Below we will we will explore the connection between ADHD and emotional regulation and how understanding this link can help individuals with ADHD manage their symptoms more effectively.

Emotional regulation refers to the ability to manage one's emotions effectively and adaptively. This involves being able to identify and understand one's own emotions, as well as those of others, and being able to regulate these emotions in a way that is appropriate for the situation. Individuals with ADHD often struggle with emotional regulation, which can make it difficult for them to manage their impulses and respond appropriately in social situations.

There are several reasons why individuals with ADHD may struggle with emotional regulation. One factor is that the same part of the brain that is responsible for attention and executive functioning (the prefrontal cortex) is also involved in emotional regulation. This means that individuals with ADHD may have difficulty regulating their emotions because their prefrontal cortex is not functioning as effectively as it should be.

Additionally, individuals with ADHD often experience heightened emotions, which can make it difficult for them to regulate their emotional responses. This is due in part to differences in brain chemistry; individuals with ADHD have been found to have lower levels of dopamine and norepinephrine, which are neurotransmitters that play a role in regulating emotions.

Finally, individuals with ADHD may struggle with emotional regulation due to past experiences of rejection or criticism. Research has found that individuals with ADHD are more likely to experience rejection and negative feedback from peers and authority figures, which can lead to feelings of shame, guilt, and low self-esteem. These negative emotions can then make it even more difficult for individuals with ADHD to regulate their emotions effectively.

Given the challenges associated with emotional regulation in individuals with ADHD, it is important to develop strategies to help manage these symptoms. One effective approach is to develop mindfulness practices, which can help individuals with ADHD become more aware of their emotional responses and learn to regulate them more effectively.

Mindfulness involves paying attention to the present moment, without judgment. This can help individuals with ADHD become more aware of their emotional responses and develop a greater understanding of how their thoughts and feelings influence their behavior. Mindfulness can also help individuals with ADHD develop greater self-compassion and reduce feelings of shame and guilt, which can be particularly important for those who have experienced rejection or criticism in the past.

Another effective strategy for managing emotional regulation in individuals with ADHD is cognitive-behavioral therapy (CBT). CBT is a type of talk therapy that focuses on changing negative thought patterns and behaviors. This can be particularly effective for individuals with ADHD who struggle with impulsivity and may benefit from learning how to identify negative thought patterns and replace them with more positive, adaptive ones.

Exercise and physical activity can also be beneficial for individuals with ADHD who struggle with emotional regulation. Regular exercise has been found to increase levels of dopamine and norepinephrine, which are neurotransmitters that play a role in regulating emotions. Exercise can also help individuals with ADHD reduce stress and improve their overall mood, which can make it easier to regulate their emotions effectively.

Finally, it is important for individuals with ADHD to develop a strong support system that includes family, friends, and mental health professionals. A strong support system can provide individuals with ADHD with the tools they need to manage their symptoms effectively, as well as emotional support during difficult times.

Strategies for managing intense emotions and mood swings

Attention-deficit/hyperactivity disorder (ADHD) is a neurodevelopmental disorder that can have a significant impact on an individual's emotional regulation. People with ADHD may struggle with impulsivity, hyperactivity, and inattention, which can lead to difficulties in managing intense emotions and mood swings. However, there are strategies that individuals with ADHD can use to manage their emotions effectively.

One important step is to increase awareness of one's emotions. Individuals with ADHD may have a tendency to react impulsively to their emotions, rather than taking the time to process them. By practicing mindfulness and tuning into their emotions, individuals with ADHD can develop a greater understanding of their emotional patterns and learn to recognize the early warning signs of an emotional outburst.

Another effective strategy is to develop coping skills that can be used in the moment. This might involve taking deep breaths, engaging in physical activity, or practicing relaxation techniques. Engaging in activities that promote relaxation and calmness, such as yoga or meditation, can also be helpful in managing intense emotions.

In addition to these individual strategies, it is important for individuals with ADHD to build a support network. This might include family, friends, or a therapist who can provide emotional support and guidance.

Group therapy or support groups can also be helpful in providing a sense of community and understanding for individuals with ADHD.

It is important to note that managing emotions is not a one-size-fits-all approach, and what works for one person may not work for another. Individuals with ADHD may need to try different strategies and techniques before finding what works best for them.

It is also important to address any underlying mental health issues that may be contributing to emotional dysregulation. For example, individuals with ADHD may also experience depression, anxiety, or other mood disorders. By treating these co-occurring conditions, individuals with ADHD can improve their overall emotional well-being.

In conclusion, emotional regulation is an important aspect of managing ADHD. By increasing awareness of one's emotions, developing coping skills, building a support network, and addressing any underlying mental health issues, individuals with ADHD can learn to effectively manage their emotions and improve their overall quality of life.

The role of therapy in improving emotional regulation

The symptoms of Attention Deficit Hyperactivity Disorder (ADHD) not only affect an individual's ability to concentrate and focus, but they can also interfere with their ability to regulate their emotions. Emotional dysregulation can be characterized by intense emotions, mood swings, difficulty controlling impulses, and difficulty with social interactions. The challenges of emotional regulation can often lead to difficulties in relationships, and it can have a significant impact on the overall quality of life. Therapy can be a helpful tool in managing these challenges and improving emotional regulation in individuals with ADHD.

One common approach to therapy for ADHD is cognitive-behavioral therapy (CBT). CBT focuses on the connection between thoughts, emotions, and behaviors. It aims to identify and challenge negative thought patterns and beliefs that can contribute to emotional dysregulation. CBT can also help individuals develop coping strategies to manage intense emotions and improve impulse control.

Another approach to therapy that has been shown to be effective in managing ADHD and improving emotional regulation is dialectical behavior therapy (DBT). DBT was originally developed to treat individuals with borderline personality disorder, but it has also been adapted for individuals with ADHD. DBT emphasizes mindfulness, distress tolerance, emotion regulation, and interpersonal effectiveness. It teaches individuals how to observe and accept their emotions without judgment, regulate their emotions, and communicate more effectively in their relationships.

In addition to therapy, there are other strategies and tools that can help individuals with ADHD improve their emotional regulation. One such strategy is exercise. Exercise has been shown to improve mood and reduce stress and anxiety. It can also increase the production of endorphins, which are chemicals in the brain that promote feelings of pleasure and well-being. Regular exercise can help individuals with ADHD feel calmer and more relaxed, which can improve emotional regulation.

Another helpful tool for improving emotional regulation in individuals with ADHD is mindfulness meditation. Mindfulness meditation involves focusing one's attention on the present moment without judgment. It can help individuals become more aware of their thoughts and emotions and learn to observe them without reacting to them. Mindfulness meditation has been shown to reduce stress, anxiety, and depression and improve emotional regulation in individuals with ADHD.

Finally, improving sleep habits can also have a positive impact on emotional regulation in individuals with ADHD. Sleep plays a crucial role in emotional regulation, and lack of sleep can contribute to emotional dysregulation. It is important for individuals with ADHD to establish a regular sleep routine and ensure that they are getting enough sleep each night.

In conclusion, emotional dysregulation is a common challenge for individuals with ADHD. Therapy, particularly cognitive-behavioral therapy and dialectical behavior therapy, can be helpful in managing these challenges and improving emotional regulation. In addition to therapy, exercise, mindfulness meditation, and improving sleep habits can also be effective tools for improving emotional regulation. By incorporating these strategies into their daily routines, individuals with ADHD can improve their overall quality of life and enhance their relationships with others.

Chapter Twenty-Seven

ADHD and Sleep

Attention-deficit/hyperactivity disorder (ADHD) is a neurological condition that affects people of all ages. Individuals with ADHD often experience challenges with attention, impulsivity, and hyperactivity, which can significantly impact their daily lives. One of the common challenges experienced by people with ADHD is sleep-related difficulties. Below we will we will explore the connection between ADHD and sleep, the types of sleep-related problems associated with ADHD, and strategies for improving sleep hygiene.

The relationship between ADHD and sleep has been widely studied, and research suggests that individuals with ADHD are at a higher risk of developing sleep problems than the general population. The prevalence of sleep disorders among individuals with ADHD is estimated to be between 50% and 70%, compared to 10% to 30% in the general population. Studies have shown that ADHD symptoms such as impulsivity, hyperactivity, and inattention can impact sleep onset, quality, and duration, leading to sleep deprivation and other health problems.

There are several types of sleep problems associated with ADHD, including insomnia, restless leg syndrome (RLS), sleep apnea, circadian rhythm disorders, and delayed sleep phase syndrome. Insomnia is the most common sleep disorder experienced by people with ADHD, characterized by difficulty falling or staying asleep. Restless leg syndrome is a neurological disorder that causes an urge to move the legs, making it difficult to sleep.

Sleep apnea is a condition that causes breathing disruptions during sleep, leading to daytime sleepiness, fatigue, and other health problems. Circadian rhythm disorders and delayed sleep phase syndrome are caused by an irregular sleep-wake cycle, making it difficult to fall asleep at night and waking up in the morning.

Improving sleep hygiene is an essential strategy for managing sleep-related problems in individuals with ADHD. Sleep hygiene refers to habits and practices that promote healthy and consistent sleep patterns. Some effective strategies for improving sleep hygiene in individuals with ADHD include establishing a consistent sleep schedule, creating a sleep-conducive environment, limiting caffeine and sugar intake, reducing screen time before bed, and engaging in relaxation techniques such as meditation and deep breathing exercises.

Therapeutic interventions can also be helpful in improving sleep-related difficulties in individuals with ADHD. Cognitive-behavioral therapy (CBT) is a commonly used therapeutic approach that has been shown to be effective in treating insomnia and other sleep-related problems. CBT aims to change negative thought patterns and behaviors related to sleep, promote relaxation, and improve sleep hygiene. In addition to CBT, other interventions such as medication, light therapy, and biofeedback may also be helpful in treating sleep problems in individuals with ADHD.

In conclusion, sleep problems are common in individuals with ADHD, and they can significantly impact their daily lives. Improving sleep hygiene through lifestyle changes such as establishing a consistent sleep schedule, creating a sleep-conducive environment, limiting caffeine and sugar intake, reducing screen time before bed, and engaging in relaxation techniques can help manage sleep-related problems in individuals with ADHD. Therapeutic interventions such as cognitive-behavioral therapy, medication, light therapy, and biofeedback can also be helpful in treating sleep problems in individuals with ADHD. It is important for individuals with ADHD to work closely with their healthcare providers to develop a comprehensive treatment plan that addresses both their ADHD symptoms and sleep-related difficulties.

The impact of ADHD on sleep patterns and quality

Attention Deficit Hyperactivity Disorder (ADHD) is a neurodevelopmental condition that affects individuals of all ages, although it is commonly diagnosed during childhood. One of the most commonly reported symptoms of ADHD is difficulty sleeping, with studies suggesting that approximately 50-70% of individuals with ADHD experience sleep problems. The relationship between ADHD and sleep is complex and can vary from person to person. Below we will we will explore the impact of ADHD on sleep patterns and quality, and discuss potential strategies for managing sleep-related challenges associated with ADHD.

Firstly, let's discuss how ADHD affects sleep patterns. Individuals with ADHD often struggle with hyperactivity, impulsivity, and racing thoughts, all of which can make it difficult to relax and fall asleep. Furthermore, many individuals with ADHD also have a delayed sleep phase, meaning they naturally stay up later and have difficulty waking up in the morning. This can lead to a vicious cycle of sleep deprivation, as individuals with ADHD may struggle to fall asleep at night and then struggle to wake up in the morning, leading to excessive daytime sleepiness and fatigue.

In addition to difficulties falling and staying asleep, individuals with ADHD also tend to have more fragmented sleep patterns, meaning they wake up more frequently throughout the night. This can lead to a decrease in the amount of deep sleep and REM sleep, which are essential for restorative and restful sleep. As a result, individuals with ADHD may wake up feeling tired and groggy, even after a full night's sleep.

The impact of ADHD on sleep quality can have significant consequences for individuals' overall health and well-being. Chronic sleep deprivation has been linked to a wide range of physical and mental health problems, including obesity, diabetes, heart disease, depression, and anxiety. Additionally, sleep deprivation can exacerbate ADHD symptoms, including inattention, hyperactivity, and impulsivity, making it even more challenging to manage daily tasks and responsibilities.

So, what can individuals with ADHD do to improve their sleep quality and manage sleep-related challenges? Firstly, it is essential to establish healthy sleep habits and routines. This may include setting a regular bedtime and wake-up time, creating a calming bedtime routine, and limiting screen time before bed. Additionally, individuals with ADHD may benefit from practicing relaxation techniques, such as meditation or deep breathing, to help calm racing thoughts and promote relaxation before bed.

Another potential strategy for managing sleep-related challenges associated with ADHD is the use of medication. Stimulant medications, such as Ritalin or Adderall, which are commonly prescribed to manage ADHD symptoms, can also improve sleep quality by reducing hyperactivity and impulsivity. However, it is important to work closely with a healthcare provider to determine the appropriate medication and dosage, as some individuals may experience sleep disturbances as a side effect of medication.

Lastly, cognitive-behavioral therapy (CBT) has been shown to be an effective treatment for improving sleep quality in individuals with ADHD. CBT for insomnia (CBT-I) is a specific type of therapy that focuses on identifying and addressing unhelpful thoughts and behaviors that may be contributing to sleep difficulties. For individuals with ADHD, this may include addressing racing thoughts and learning relaxation techniques to help promote sleep.

In conclusion, sleep problems are a common challenge for individuals with ADHD, with approximately 50-70% of individuals with ADHD experiencing sleep difficulties. ADHD can impact sleep quality by making it difficult to relax and fall asleep, leading to a vicious cycle of sleep deprivation and fatigue. However, there are strategies for managing sleep-related challenges associated with ADHD, including establishing healthy sleep habits and routines, medication, and cognitive-behavioral therapy. By prioritizing sleep and developing effective strategies for managing sleep-related challenges, individuals with ADHD can improve their overall health and well-being.

Strategies for improving sleep hygiene and addressing sleep disorders

Sleep is essential for physical and mental health, but individuals with attention deficit hyperactivity disorder (ADHD) often struggle with sleep-related issues. ADHD can interfere with the ability to fall asleep and stay asleep, leading to chronic sleep deprivation and other health problems. Below we will we will discuss the impact of ADHD on sleep patterns and quality, and strategies for improving sleep hygiene and addressing sleep disorders.

The Impact of ADHD on Sleep

Individuals with ADHD are more likely to experience sleep-related issues than those without the condition. According to a study, up to 70% of children and 80% of adults with ADHD experience sleep disturbances. These disturbances can take many forms, such as difficulty falling asleep, staying asleep, or waking up too early.

One of the main reasons for these issues is that individuals with ADHD have an overactive mind, which makes it hard to relax and fall asleep. In addition, the symptoms of ADHD, such as impulsivity and hyperactivity, can interfere with sleep as well. Individuals with ADHD may struggle to maintain a regular sleep schedule or avoid stimulating activities before bedtime, leading to poor sleep hygiene.

Sleep disturbances can have a significant impact on an individual's daily life. Chronic sleep deprivation can lead to fatigue, irritability, and poor concentration, all of which can exacerbate the symptoms of ADHD. Lack of sleep can also lead to other health problems, such as obesity, diabetes, and cardiovascular disease.

Strategies for Improving Sleep Hygiene

Improving sleep hygiene is essential for individuals with ADHD to address their sleep-related issues. Here are some strategies that can help:

1. Establish a consistent sleep schedule: Going to bed and waking up at the same time every day can help regulate the body's internal clock and promote better sleep.

2. Create a relaxing bedtime routine: Engage in relaxing activities before bedtime, such as taking a warm bath, reading a book, or practicing meditation. This can help calm the mind and prepare the body for sleep.

3. Avoid stimulating activities before bedtime: Avoid activities that can interfere with sleep, such as using electronic devices, watching television, or exercising.

4. Create a comfortable sleep environment: Make sure the bedroom is quiet, dark, and cool. Use comfortable bedding and a supportive mattress to promote restful sleep.

5. Limit caffeine and alcohol consumption: Caffeine and alcohol can interfere with sleep, so it's important to limit consumption before bedtime.

Addressing Sleep Disorders

In some cases, individuals with ADHD may also have sleep disorders that require medical intervention. Some common sleep disorders that can co-occur with ADHD include:

6. Insomnia: Insomnia is a sleep disorder characterized by difficulty falling or staying asleep. Individuals with ADHD may have trouble quieting their minds at bedtime, leading to insomnia.

7. Sleep Apnea: Sleep apnea is a sleep disorder characterized by interrupted breathing during sleep. Individuals with ADHD may be at a higher risk for sleep apnea due to hyperactivity and impulsivity.

8. Restless Leg Syndrome: Restless leg syndrome is a sleep disorder characterized by uncomfortable sensations in the legs, which can lead to difficulty falling asleep or staying asleep. Individuals with ADHD may be at a higher risk for restless leg syndrome due to sensory processing issues.

Treatment for these sleep disorders may include medication, therapy, or lifestyle modifications. It's essential to work with a healthcare professional to determine the best course of treatment for each individual.

The role of sleep in overall ADHD management

Attention Deficit Hyperactivity Disorder (ADHD) is a neurodevelopmental disorder that affects people of all ages. One of the most common challenges that people with ADHD face is difficulty sleeping. Research has shown that people with ADHD have higher rates of sleep disturbances and disorders, such as insomnia, restless leg syndrome, and sleep apnea, than the general population. Below we will we will explore the impact of sleep on ADHD and the importance of managing sleep for overall ADHD management.

People with ADHD often experience difficulty falling asleep, staying asleep, and waking up in the morning. These sleep disturbances can lead to excessive daytime sleepiness, fatigue, irritability, and difficulty concentrating. For people with ADHD, the lack of sleep can exacerbate their symptoms, making it even more difficult to focus, stay organized, and manage their emotions.

Research has also shown that sleep deprivation can affect the brain functions that are essential for managing ADHD symptoms. Sleep deprivation can lead to impaired cognitive functions, such as working memory, attention, and impulse control, which are already challenging for people with ADHD. As a result, lack of sleep can worsen ADHD symptoms and interfere with treatment progress.

Therefore, it is crucial for people with ADHD to prioritize sleep hygiene and develop healthy sleep habits to manage their symptoms effectively. The following are some strategies for improving sleep hygiene and addressing sleep disorders:

1. Establish a consistent sleep routine: Go to bed and wake up at the same time every day, even on weekends. Establishing a consistent sleep routine helps regulate the body's internal clock and promotes better sleep quality.

2. Create a sleep-conducive environment: Make sure your bedroom is dark, quiet, and cool. Avoid using electronic devices, such as smartphones or laptops, in bed, as the blue light emitted by these devices can interfere with sleep quality.

3. Avoid caffeine, alcohol, and nicotine: These substances can disrupt sleep and affect the quality of sleep.

4. Exercise regularly: Regular physical activity can help regulate the sleep-wake cycle and promote better sleep quality.

5. Cognitive-behavioral therapy (CBT): CBT is a form of talk therapy that helps people with ADHD identify and change negative thought patterns and behaviors that interfere with sleep. CBT can be helpful for people with insomnia and other sleep disorders.

6. Medication: In some cases, medication may be necessary to manage sleep disorders, such as sleep apnea or restless leg syndrome.

In addition to managing sleep hygiene, it is essential for people with ADHD to work with their healthcare providers to develop a comprehensive treatment plan that addresses their symptoms and individual needs. Treatment for ADHD often includes a combination of medication, therapy, and lifestyle modifications, such as exercise and diet changes.

In conclusion, sleep plays a crucial role in managing ADHD symptoms, and sleep disturbances can exacerbate the challenges that people with ADHD face. Therefore, it is essential for people with ADHD to prioritize sleep hygiene and develop healthy sleep habits to manage their symptoms effectively. By working with their healthcare providers and following evidence-based strategies, people with ADHD can improve their sleep quality and overall well-being.

Chapter Twenty-Eight

Self-Advocacy and Empowerment

Self-advocacy and empowerment are critical for individuals with ADHD to thrive in various aspects of their lives. Self-advocacy refers to the process of advocating for oneself, including the identification and communication of needs, goals, and preferences, and taking charge of one's own learning and development. Empowerment, on the other hand, involves gaining the knowledge, skills, and confidence to take control of one's life and make informed decisions that lead to positive outcomes. Below we will we will explore the importance of self-advocacy and empowerment for individuals with ADHD and provide strategies for developing these skills.

Individuals with ADHD often face challenges in academic, social, and occupational settings. However, with self-advocacy skills, they can work with their teachers, employers, and peers to communicate their needs and find solutions that work for them. For instance, a student with ADHD may need extra time on tests or assignments, prefer a quieter workspace, or require additional resources to support their learning. By advocating for themselves, they can ensure that their needs are met, and they can achieve academic success.

Similarly, in the workplace, individuals with ADHD may face challenges such as difficulty with time management, distractions, and forgetfulness. However, by advocating for themselves and communicating their needs to their employer, they can find strategies to address these challenges. For instance, they may ask for accommodations such as flexible work hours or the use of a task management system. By doing so, they can perform at their best and achieve success in their careers.

Empowerment is also critical for individuals with ADHD to achieve success and satisfaction in their lives. Empowerment involves developing a sense of control over one's life, and it can be achieved through education, support, and self-awareness. By gaining knowledge about their condition, including their strengths and challenges, individuals with ADHD can take control of their lives and make informed decisions that align with their goals.

Support is also crucial in empowering individuals with ADHD. Support may come from family, friends, or support groups, and it can provide individuals with the encouragement and resources needed to achieve their goals. For instance, support groups can provide a safe space for individuals with ADHD to share their experiences, learn from others, and develop new strategies for managing their symptoms.

Self-awareness is another critical component of empowerment. By understanding their strengths and weaknesses, individuals with ADHD can develop strategies to address their challenges and build on their strengths. Self-awareness also involves recognizing and managing emotions, which is particularly important for individuals with ADHD, who may struggle with emotional regulation. By developing strategies such as mindfulness and self-care, individuals with ADHD can take control of their emotions and improve their overall well-being.

There are several strategies that individuals with ADHD can use to develop self-advocacy and empowerment skills. These strategies include:

1. Developing a support network: Individuals with ADHD should seek out support from family, friends, or support groups. Support can provide encouragement and resources needed to achieve their goals.

2. Seeking education: Individuals with ADHD should seek knowledge about their condition, including their strengths and challenges. Education can help individuals take control of their lives and make informed decisions.

3. Developing self-awareness: Individuals with ADHD should develop self-awareness by recognizing their strengths and weaknesses, managing their emotions, and practicing self-care.

4. Developing communication skills: Effective communication is essential for self-advocacy. Individuals with ADHD should develop communication skills to express their needs and preferences.

5. Seeking accommodations: Individuals with ADHD should seek accommodations in academic, social, and occupational settings. Accommodations can help individuals achieve their goals and perform at their best.

Developing self-advocacy skills for individuals with ADHD

Attention Deficit Hyperactivity Disorder (ADHD) can pose various challenges in daily life. However, with effective self-advocacy skills, individuals with ADHD can overcome these obstacles and improve their quality of life. Self-advocacy refers to the ability to speak up for oneself and assert personal needs, preferences, and rights. Below we will we will discuss the importance of developing self-advocacy skills for individuals with ADHD and provide some strategies for doing so.

Firstly, it is important to understand why self-advocacy is crucial for individuals with ADHD. Many individuals with ADHD struggle with executive functioning, which can lead to difficulties with organization, time management, and communication. This can result in feeling misunderstood, isolated, and frustrated. By developing self-advocacy skills, individuals with ADHD can communicate their needs and preferences more effectively and advocate for themselves in various settings, including school, work, and social situations.

One important aspect of self-advocacy for individuals with ADHD is the ability to communicate their diagnosis and its impact on their daily life. Many people with ADHD may feel hesitant to disclose their diagnosis due to fear of judgment or stigma. However, by sharing their diagnosis and how it affects them, they can receive appropriate accommodations and support. This can include requesting extra time on exams or tasks, flexible work hours, or accommodations such as fidget toys or noise-cancelling headphones. It is important to remember that ADHD is a neurodevelopmental condition and that accommodations are not a sign of weakness but a means of leveling the playing field.

Another important skill for self-advocacy is the ability to recognize and communicate personal strengths and weaknesses. This involves understanding how ADHD affects one's functioning and recognizing what strategies work best for managing symptoms. For example, an individual with ADHD may benefit from using a planner, breaking down tasks into smaller steps, or taking breaks to manage their attention. By identifying and communicating these strategies to others, individuals with ADHD can better advocate for their needs and demonstrate their strengths.

Assertiveness is also a crucial component of self-advocacy. Individuals with ADHD may struggle with assertiveness due to challenges with impulse control and social communication. However, it is important to develop assertiveness skills to communicate personal boundaries, express concerns or disagreements, and advocate for oneself in a respectful and effective manner. This can involve using "I" statements to communicate personal feelings and needs, practicing active listening to better understand others' perspectives, and setting clear boundaries with others.

Finally, self-advocacy can involve seeking out and utilizing available resources and support. This can include reaching out to peer support groups, seeking therapy or coaching, or accessing online resources and tools for managing ADHD symptoms. By actively seeking out these resources and advocating for oneself, individuals with ADHD can take control of their condition and work towards achieving their goals.

In terms of specific strategies for developing self-advocacy skills, there are several things that individuals with ADHD can do to improve their ability to advocate for themselves. These include:

1. Education: Learn as much as possible about ADHD and how it affects you personally. This can help you better communicate your needs and educate others about the condition.

2. Role-Playing: Practicing assertiveness skills through role-playing scenarios can help build confidence and prepare individuals for real-life situations.

3. Build a Support System: Connect with others who understand and can relate to your experiences. This can include peer support groups or online communities.

4. Set Realistic Goals: Setting realistic goals and breaking them down into manageable steps can help build a sense of control and achievement.

5. Self-Care: Prioritizing self-care can improve overall well-being and increase resilience in the face of ADHD-related challenges.

Navigating the healthcare system and advocating for appropriate treatment

Navigating the healthcare system can be a challenge for anyone, but it can be especially difficult for individuals with ADHD. Accessing appropriate treatment and support can be a complex and overwhelming process, but it is crucial for the well-being and success of individuals with ADHD. Below we will we will explore some strategies for navigating the healthcare system and advocating for appropriate treatment for individuals with ADHD.

The first step in advocating for appropriate treatment is to educate oneself about ADHD and its symptoms. Individuals with ADHD should seek out reliable sources of information and stay up-to-date on the latest research and treatment options. This can be done through reading books, attending conferences and workshops, and consulting with healthcare professionals.

Once individuals with ADHD have a good understanding of their condition and its symptoms, they can begin to explore their treatment options. It is important to note that there is no one-size-fits-all approach to treating ADHD. What works for one individual may not work for another. However, there are several evidence-based treatments that have been shown to be effective for many individuals with ADHD.

Some of the most commonly used treatments for ADHD include medication, therapy, and lifestyle modifications. Medication can be very effective in reducing symptoms such as hyperactivity, impulsivity, and inattention. Therapy can help individuals with ADHD develop coping strategies and improve their self-esteem. Lifestyle modifications such as regular exercise, healthy eating, and good sleep hygiene can also help to improve symptoms and overall well-being.

Once individuals with ADHD have identified the treatment options that are most appropriate for their needs, they can begin to navigate the healthcare system to access those treatments. This can be a daunting process, but there are several strategies that can help.

The first step is to find a healthcare provider who specializes in treating ADHD. This may be a psychiatrist, psychologist, or other mental health professional. It is important to find a provider who is knowledgeable about ADHD and who has experience working with individuals with this condition.

Once a healthcare provider has been identified, individuals with ADHD should be prepared to advocate for themselves and their needs. This may involve asking questions about treatment options, expressing concerns about side effects or other issues, and advocating for their own preferences and priorities.

It can also be helpful for individuals with ADHD to bring a friend or family member to appointments for support and advocacy. This person can help to ask questions, provide additional information, and offer emotional support.

In addition to advocating for themselves in healthcare settings, individuals with ADHD can also advocate for their needs in other areas of life. This may include advocating for accommodations in school or at work, seeking out support groups or other resources, and being open and honest with friends and family members about their condition.

Self-advocacy is a crucial skill for individuals with ADHD to develop, as it can help to ensure that they receive the appropriate treatment and support they need to thrive. It can be a challenging and sometimes uncomfortable process, but with practice and support, individuals with ADHD can become effective advocates for their own needs and priorities.

In conclusion, navigating the healthcare system and advocating for appropriate treatment can be a complex and overwhelming process for individuals with ADHD. However, by educating oneself about the condition and treatment options, identifying a knowledgeable healthcare provider, and developing self-advocacy skills, individuals with ADHD can access the support and resources they need to manage their symptoms and achieve success in all areas of life.

Building confidence and embracing personal strengths

Attention-deficit/hyperactivity disorder (ADHD) is a neurodevelopmental disorder characterized by symptoms of inattention, hyperactivity, and impulsivity. Individuals with ADHD may face various challenges in their daily lives, including difficulty with organization, time management, and emotional regulation. However, it's important to note that individuals with ADHD also possess unique strengths and talents. Building confidence and embracing personal strengths can be a crucial aspect of managing ADHD symptoms and thriving in personal and professional settings.

One strategy for building confidence and embracing personal strengths is to focus on positive self-talk. This involves identifying and challenging negative thoughts or beliefs about oneself and replacing them with positive affirmations. For example, instead of thinking "I'm so disorganized," one could say "I'm good at coming up with creative solutions." By reframing negative self-talk in this way, individuals with ADHD can begin to shift their mindset and focus on their strengths rather than their weaknesses.

Another important aspect of building confidence and embracing personal strengths is to engage in activities that promote a sense of accomplishment and mastery. For individuals with ADHD, this may involve pursuing hobbies or interests that align with their unique talents and strengths. For example, someone who excels at visual-spatial reasoning may enjoy activities such as drawing or graphic design. Similarly, someone with a talent for music may find fulfillment in playing an instrument or singing.

It's also important for individuals with ADHD to recognize and acknowledge their successes, no matter how small they may seem. This can help to build self-esteem and reinforce positive behaviors. Keeping a journal or calendar to track accomplishments and progress can be a helpful tool in this regard.

In addition to focusing on personal strengths, it's important for individuals with ADHD to surround themselves with a supportive network of family, friends, and professionals. This can include seeking out a therapist or coach who specializes in ADHD, joining a support group, or simply confiding in trusted friends or family members. By sharing their experiences and challenges with others who understand, individuals with ADHD can feel less alone and more empowered to navigate their daily lives.

Finally, it's important for individuals with ADHD to recognize that they are not defined by their diagnosis. While ADHD can present challenges, it's important to remember that everyone has strengths and weaknesses. By embracing personal strengths and working to manage symptoms, individuals with ADHD can lead fulfilling and successful lives.

Chapter Twenty-Nine

The Role of Support Networks

The journey with ADHD can be a challenging one, and it is important to have a support network in place to help navigate these challenges. Support networks can include family members, friends, mental health professionals, and peer support groups. Below we will we will explore the role of support networks in managing ADHD.

Firstly, family members and close friends can play a significant role in supporting individuals with ADHD. They can provide emotional support, help with daily tasks, and offer a non-judgmental listening ear. It is important for family members and friends to understand the symptoms and challenges of ADHD, as well as the strengths and abilities of the individual. This understanding can help family members and friends better support the individual with ADHD.

Secondly, mental health professionals such as therapists, psychiatrists, and psychologists can play a crucial role in managing ADHD. These professionals can provide therapy, medication management, and other interventions that can help individuals with ADHD manage symptoms and improve their quality of life. Mental health professionals can also provide support for family members and friends, as they navigate the challenges of supporting someone with ADHD.

Thirdly, peer support groups can be an important resource for individuals with ADHD. These groups provide a space for individuals with ADHD to connect with others who understand their experiences and challenges.

Peer support groups can offer practical advice, emotional support, and a sense of community. Many peer support groups are available online, making them accessible to individuals who may not have access to in-person support.

In addition to these support networks, it is important for individuals with ADHD to also develop their own self-support systems. This can include self-care practices such as exercise, meditation, and healthy eating habits. It can also include self-advocacy skills, such as learning to speak up for oneself and ask for accommodations when needed.

Building a strong support network can help individuals with ADHD manage their symptoms and live fulfilling lives. It is important for individuals with ADHD to seek out support networks that work for them, and to be open to trying different options until they find the right fit. With the right support, individuals with ADHD can learn to embrace their strengths and manage their challenges with confidence.

The importance of understanding and empathy from family and friends

Attention Deficit Hyperactivity Disorder (ADHD) is a neurodevelopmental disorder that affects individuals of all ages. While there is no cure for ADHD, there are various treatments and strategies available that can help individuals manage symptoms and improve their quality of life. One of the most important factors in managing ADHD is having a strong support network, particularly from family and friends.

ADHD can often be misunderstood and stigmatized, leading to negative attitudes and perceptions towards those who live with the condition. This can be especially challenging for children and adolescents, who may be subject to bullying or social exclusion. It is crucial that family members and friends take the time to understand what ADHD is and how it affects their loved one. This understanding can lead to increased empathy and a more positive attitude towards the individual, which can have a significant impact on their self-esteem and overall well-being.

In addition to understanding and empathy, family and friends can provide practical support to individuals with ADHD. This can include helping to establish and maintain routines, setting reminders, and providing a structured and organized environment. For children with ADHD, this can be particularly important in helping them to develop good habits and routines that will benefit them throughout their lives.

It is also important for family and friends to recognize and celebrate the strengths and talents of individuals with ADHD. While individuals with ADHD may struggle with certain tasks, they often have unique strengths and abilities that should be recognized and nurtured. For example, individuals with ADHD may be highly creative, have a great sense of humor, or be able to think outside the box. Recognizing and celebrating these strengths can help to boost self-esteem and foster a positive sense of identity.

In addition to support from family and friends, individuals with ADHD may benefit from joining support groups or seeking out therapy. Support groups can provide a sense of community and connection with others who are experiencing similar challenges, while therapy can help individuals develop strategies for managing symptoms and improving their quality of life.

It is important to note that support from family and friends should not be a substitute for professional treatment. ADHD is a complex condition that can have significant impacts on an individual's life, and professional treatment is often necessary to manage symptoms effectively. However, having a strong support network can be a valuable complement to professional treatment, helping individuals to feel more supported and empowered as they navigate the challenges of living with ADHD.

In conclusion, the role of family and friends in supporting individuals with ADHD is crucial. Understanding and empathy can go a long way in helping individuals with ADHD feel accepted and supported, while practical support and recognition of strengths can help to boost self-esteem and foster a positive sense of identity. Joining support groups and seeking out therapy can also be helpful in managing symptoms and improving quality of life. By working together and providing a strong support network, family and friends can play an important role in helping individuals with ADHD to thrive.

Accessing professional support and resources

ADHD (Attention Deficit Hyperactivity Disorder) is a complex neurodevelopmental disorder that affects approximately 6-7% of children and 2-3% of adults worldwide. While ADHD can pose significant challenges for those living with it, accessing appropriate professional support and resources can help individuals with ADHD lead fulfilling and productive lives. Below we will we will discuss the importance of accessing professional support and resources for individuals with ADHD and their families.

The first step in accessing professional support and resources for individuals with ADHD is to get an accurate diagnosis from a qualified healthcare professional. A diagnosis of ADHD involves a comprehensive evaluation of a person's symptoms, medical history, and behavioral patterns. Once a diagnosis is made, a healthcare professional can recommend appropriate treatment and support services. It is essential to seek out healthcare professionals with experience in diagnosing and treating ADHD to ensure that individuals receive the best possible care.

One of the most effective treatments for ADHD is medication. There are several types of medications available to treat ADHD, including stimulants and non-stimulants. Stimulant medications are the most commonly prescribed medication for ADHD and are typically prescribed for children aged six years and older, adolescents, and adults. Non-stimulant medications may be prescribed for individuals who cannot tolerate stimulant medications or have other medical conditions that make stimulant medications unsuitable. While medication is an essential part of ADHD treatment, it is not a cure-all and should be used in conjunction with other support services.

Another important support service for individuals with ADHD is therapy. Therapy can help individuals with ADHD develop coping strategies and learn skills to manage symptoms, such as impulsivity, distractibility, and hyperactivity. There are several types of therapy that can be effective in treating ADHD, including cognitive-behavioral therapy, family therapy, and social skills training. Cognitive-behavioral therapy helps individuals with ADHD understand the relationship between their thoughts, feelings, and behaviors, and teaches them how to modify their behavior to better manage symptoms. Family therapy can help families better understand ADHD and develop strategies to support their loved one with ADHD. Social skills training can help individuals with ADHD improve their communication and interpersonal skills, which can be challenging for those with the disorder.

In addition to medication and therapy, there are several other support services that can be helpful for individuals with ADHD. For children with ADHD, early intervention programs, such as early childhood education and behavior therapy, can help manage symptoms and improve outcomes. Educational support services, such as special education and academic accommodations, can help children with ADHD succeed in school.

Vocational rehabilitation services can help adults with ADHD find and maintain employment. Support groups can also be helpful for individuals with ADHD and their families, providing a sense of community and a safe space to share experiences and coping strategies.

It is essential to note that accessing professional support and resources for individuals with ADHD is not always straightforward. There are significant barriers to accessing care, including financial barriers, lack of access to specialized healthcare providers, and stigma. Many individuals with ADHD face financial barriers to care, including high medication costs and limited insurance coverage for mental health services. Additionally, there is a shortage of healthcare providers with specialized training in diagnosing and treating ADHD, particularly in rural areas. Finally, there is a significant stigma surrounding ADHD and other mental health disorders, which can make it difficult for individuals to seek out care and support.

In conclusion, accessing professional support and resources is crucial for individuals with ADHD and their families. An accurate diagnosis, medication, therapy, and other support services can help individuals with ADHD manage symptoms and lead fulfilling lives. However, significant barriers to accessing care exist, including financial barriers, lack of access to specialized healthcare providers, and stigma. It is essential to address these barriers and increase access to care for individuals with ADHD to improve outcomes and reduce the burden of the disorder

Summing up key takeaways from the book

As we come to the end of this book on ADHD, it's important to reflect on the key takeaways and lessons that can be learned from it. ADHD is a complex and multifaceted condition that affects millions of people around the world, and it can be challenging to navigate for both individuals living with ADHD and their loved ones.

One of the most important things to understand about ADHD is that it is not a choice or a character flaw. It is a neurodevelopmental disorder that affects the brain's ability to regulate attention, behavior, and emotions. This can lead to a range of symptoms, including difficulty with focus, impulsivity, hyperactivity, and emotional dysregulation.

However, it's also important to recognize that ADHD can come with unique strengths and abilities. Many individuals with ADHD are highly creative, innovative, and energetic, and they can excel in areas that require out-of-the-box thinking and spontaneity.

Throughout this book, we've explored a range of topics related to ADHD, from understanding the basics of the condition and its symptoms to learning about the latest research and treatment options. We've also discussed strategies for improving time management and organization, addressing sleep disorders, developing self-advocacy skills, and building a support network.

One of the most important themes that has emerged throughout this book is the importance of mindfulness and self-compassion. Living with ADHD can be challenging, and it's easy to get caught up in feelings of shame, guilt, and frustration. However, by practicing mindfulness and self-compassion, individuals with ADHD can learn to accept themselves and their struggles and build a sense of inner resilience and strength.

Another key takeaway from this book is the importance of seeking professional help when needed. ADHD is a treatable condition, and there are a range of evidence-based treatments available, including medication, therapy, and lifestyle interventions. By working with healthcare professionals and taking a comprehensive approach to treatment, individuals with ADHD can improve their symptoms and overall quality of life.

In addition to seeking professional help, it's also important for individuals with ADHD to build a strong support network of family, friends, and peers. Having a supportive community can help to reduce feelings of isolation and provide emotional and practical support when needed.

Finally, it's important to remember that living with ADHD is a journey, and there will be ups and downs along the way. However, with the right tools, strategies, and support, individuals with ADHD can learn to manage their symptoms and lead fulfilling and successful lives.

In conclusion, this book has provided a comprehensive and informative overview of ADHD and its impact on individuals and their families. By embracing a compassionate and open-minded approach, and by seeking out evidence-based treatments and support, individuals with ADHD can learn to thrive and succeed in all areas of life.

Emphasizing the importance of continued learning and growth

In recent years, there has been a growing emphasis on the importance of continued learning and growth, particularly for individuals with ADHD. This is because ADHD is a complex disorder that can have a significant impact on various aspects of life, including academic performance, career success, and personal relationships. Therefore, it is essential for individuals with ADHD to develop strategies and skills that can help them overcome their challenges and achieve their goals.

One of the most important strategies for continued learning and growth for individuals with ADHD is self-awareness. This involves understanding one's strengths and weaknesses, as well as recognizing the symptoms of ADHD and how they can impact daily life. By increasing self-awareness, individuals with ADHD can better identify their specific needs and develop strategies to manage their symptoms.

Another critical aspect of continued learning and growth is education. Individuals with ADHD can benefit greatly from learning about the disorder, including its causes, symptoms, and treatment options. This can help them to better understand their condition and to develop strategies that can help them manage their symptoms.

Additionally, individuals with ADHD can benefit from learning new skills and techniques that can help them overcome their challenges. For example, cognitive-behavioral therapy (CBT) is a type of psychotherapy that has been shown to be effective in helping individuals with ADHD develop coping strategies and improve their executive functioning skills. Similarly, mindfulness meditation has been found to be an effective tool for managing ADHD-related symptoms such as impulsivity and hyperactivity.

In addition to these strategies, it is also important for individuals with ADHD to develop a support system. This can include family, friends, and healthcare professionals who can provide guidance and encouragement. It is also helpful to connect with others who have ADHD and share similar experiences. This can be achieved through support groups or online communities.

Finally, it is important for individuals with ADHD to continue to seek out new opportunities for growth and development. This can involve pursuing higher education, learning a new skill or hobby, or seeking out new experiences that can challenge and stimulate the mind.

In conclusion, continued learning and growth is crucial for individuals with ADHD. By increasing self-awareness, educating themselves about the disorder, and learning new skills and techniques, individuals with ADHD can develop strategies that can help them overcome their challenges and achieve their goals. Additionally, by building a support system and seeking out new opportunities for growth and development, individuals with ADHD can lead fulfilling and successful lives.

Encouragement for the journey ahead in managing ADHD

Attention-deficit/hyperactivity disorder (ADHD) can present numerous challenges in various aspects of life, including education, work, relationships, and overall quality of life. However, it is important to remember that managing ADHD is a journey that requires patience, dedication, and a willingness to learn and grow. While there may be setbacks and frustrations along the way, there are also many strategies and resources available to help individuals with ADHD thrive.

One of the most important factors in managing ADHD is taking an active role in one's own treatment and seeking out appropriate resources and support. This may include working with a healthcare provider to develop a treatment plan that includes medication, therapy, and lifestyle changes, as well as utilizing resources such as support groups, educational materials, and online forums. It is important to remember that there is no one-size-fits-all approach to managing ADHD, and what works for one person may not work for another. Therefore, it is important to remain open to trying new strategies and approaches, and to be willing to adjust as needed.

Another important aspect of managing ADHD is building a support network of family, friends, and healthcare providers who understand and can offer encouragement and assistance. This may include seeking out a therapist or coach who specializes in ADHD, joining a support group or online community, and educating family and friends about the disorder and how it affects daily life. It is important to remember that seeking help is a sign of strength, not weakness, and that there is no shame in needing support.

Additionally, it is important to focus on building self-awareness and developing strategies for managing symptoms in various areas of life. This may include developing habits and routines that promote organization and time management, utilizing mindfulness practices to manage emotions and improve focus, and seeking out resources and accommodations in academic and work settings. It is also important to recognize and embrace personal strengths and talents, and to focus on building self-confidence and resilience in the face of challenges.

Finally, it is important to remember that managing ADHD is a continuous process that requires ongoing learning and growth. While there may be times when progress seems slow or setbacks occur, it is important to remain committed to the journey and to keep moving forward. This may involve seeking out new resources and strategies, working with healthcare providers to adjust treatment plans, and focusing on developing new skills and habits.

In conclusion, managing ADHD can be a challenging journey, but it is also a journey that offers opportunities for growth, learning, and self-discovery. By taking an active role in one's own treatment, building a supportive network of family and friends, developing effective strategies for managing symptoms, and embracing a mindset of continuous learning and growth, individuals with ADHD can thrive and achieve their goals.

SD - #0029 - 140926 - C0 - 229/152/15 - PB - 9781776969241 - Matt Lamination